Vital Notes for Nurses: Promoting Health

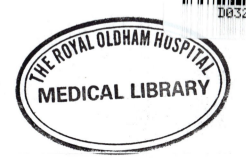

Vital Notes for Nurses are indispensable guides for student nurses taking the pre-registration programme in all branches of nursing.

These concise, accessible books assume no prior knowledge. Each book in the series clearly presents the essential facts in context in a user-friendly format and provides students and qualified nurses with a thorough understanding of the core topics which inform professional practice.

Published

Vital Notes for Nurses: Psychology
Sue Barker
ISBN: 978-1-405-1-5520-5

Vital Notes for Nurses: Accountability
Helen Caulfield
ISBN: 978-1-4051-2279-5

Vital Notes for Nurses: Health Assessment
Edited by Anna Crouch and Clency Meurier
ISBN: 978-1-4051-1458-5

Vital Notes for Nurses: Professional Development, Reflection and Decision-making
Melanie Jasper
ISBN: 978-1-4051-3261-9

Vital Notes for Nurses: Nursing Theory
Hugh McKenna and Oliver Slevin
ISBN: 978-1-4051-3702-7

Vital Notes for Nurses: Research for Evidence-Based Practice
Robert Newell and Philip Burnard
ISBN: 978-1-4051-2562-9

Vital Notes for Nurses: Principles of Care
Hilary Lloyd
ISBN: 978-1-4051-4598-5

Vital Notes for Nurses: Promoting Health
Jane Wills
ISBN: 978-1-4051-3999-1

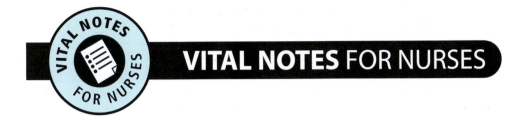

VITAL NOTES FOR NURSES

Promoting Health

Edited by
Jane Wills

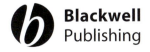

Blackwell
Publishing

© 2007 by Blackwell Publishing Ltd.

Blackwell Publishing editorial offices:
Blackwell Publishing Ltd, 9600 Garsington Road, Oxford OX4 2DQ, UK
Tel: +44 (0)1865 776868
Blackwell Publishing Inc., 350 Main Street, Malden, MA 02148-5020, USA
Tel: +1 781 388 8250
Blackwell Publishing Asia Pty Ltd, 550 Swanston Street, Carlton, Victoria
3053, Australia
Tel: +61 (0)3 8359 1011

First published 2007 by Blackwell Publishing Ltd

ISBN: 978-1-4051-3999-1

Library of Congress Cataloging-in-Publication Data

Promoting health / edited by Jane Wills.
p. ; cm. – (Vital notes for nurses)
Includes bibliographical references and index.
ISBN-13: 978-1-4051-3999-1 (pbk. : alk. paper)
ISBN-10: 1-4051-3999-4 (pbk. : alk. paper)
1. Public health nursing. 2. Health promotion.
I. Wills, Jane, MSc. II. Series.
[DNLM: 1. Health Promotion. 2. Public Health Nursing–
methods. 3. Nurse's Role. 4. Nurse-Patient Relations. 5. Patient
Education. WY 108 P965 2007]
RT97.P76 2007
613–dc22
2006100266

A catalogue record for this title is available from the British Library

Set in 10/12 Palatino
by SNP Best-set Typesetter Ltd., Hong Kong
Printed and bound in Singapore
by COS Printers Pte Ltd

The publisher's policy is to use permanent paper from mills that operate a
sustainable forestry policy, and which has been manufactured from pulp
processed using acid-free and elementary chlorine-free practices.
Furthermore, the publisher ensures that the text paper and cover board used
have met acceptable environmental accreditation standards.

For further information on Blackwell Publishing, visit our website:
www.blackwellnursing.com

Contents

Preface

Health is everybody's business. We have a population that is living longer and is likely to carry a burden of chronic disease. An increasing number of products, treatments and information are available to an informed health consumer and 'health' is discussed by those as diverse as Kylie Minogue in relation to breast cancer, Jamie Oliver in relation to healthy food for children and Bill Gates in relation to human immunodeficiency virus/acquired immune deficiency syndrome (HIV/AIDS) treatments. Globalisation means the worldwide spread and movement not only of products but also people (including health sector workers) and diseases. Better population health depends on making health everybody's business but nurses have a vital role to play. As key health professionals, you are in a unique position to act as powerful advocates for a future healthy planet; to ensure equity particularly in access to health care and services; and to make the healthy choice the easier choice. Nurses make a major difference across the life cycle and in their commitment to vulnerable or marginalised groups, such as the poor, the elderly, refugees and asylum seekers, and the homeless. This book is about protecting the health of the public by preventing disease and illness particularly through identifying risk and promoting health by supporting and maintaining a healthier lifestyle and the building of healthier communities. These are probably the most important parts of your nursing role. Health matters – it is a human right and it is sound economic investment.

Jane Wills

About the Authors

Amanda Hesman is Senior Lecturer Adult Nursing at London South Bank University where she teaches Public Health. She is a registered nurse with a particular interest in sexual and reproductive health and has worked as a health advisor in genitourinary medicine (GUM) in Brighton and as a GUM researcher in London. She has an MA in Women's Studies and is a member of the UK Public Health Association and British Association of Sexual Health and HIV.

Jenny Husbands is Senior Lecturer Adult Nursing at London South Bank University where she teaches Public Health. She has worked as a health visitor and has also worked in a Health Promotion department with responsibility for working with primary care organisations and practitioners. She is also a keep fit teacher.

Linda Jackson is currently Health Development Manager for Greenwich Primary Care Trust. Prior to this she was Senior Lecturer in the MSC Public Health/Health Promotion degree programme at London South Bank University. She has also taught in the School of Public Health at Curtin University in Western Australia and worked in a variety of posts in Australia and the USA. Her primary interests are in nutrition, health promotion practice and workforce development.

Susie Sykes is Senior Lecturer in Public Health and Health Promotion at London South Bank University. She has worked in public health for ten years having worked in the voluntary sector prior to that. Her professional practice interests are work with young people, community development and in recent years public health evaluation. Susie combines an academic career with freelance work in strategy development and project evaluation mostly for public sector organisations.

Jane Wills is Reader in Public Health and Health Promotion at London South Bank University. She has written extensively on health promotion and been influential in its development as a field of activity over the past 20 years. Her textbooks have been translated into five languages and are on the core curricula of nursing and health studies in many countries. She is co-editor of *Critical Public Health*, an international peer-reviewed journal dedicated to critical analyses of theory and practice, reviews of the literature and explorations of new ways of working. She has a visiting Professorship at the University of Witwatersrand in Johannesburg where she works with primary health care workers and researchers on HIV/AIDS, nutrition and other public health issues.

Introduction: The Role of the Nurse in Promoting Health

Jane Wills

Introduction

This book is intended to clarify for new nurses the importance of developing public health and health promotion skills. Developing such skills demands a wide range of knowledge, drawing from the scientific knowledge of epidemiology to an understanding of health policy to communication skills. Such knowledge must then be applied to the needs of the individual, family, group, community or population and because the National Health Service (NHS) is not the only sector that affects and is concerned with health, the nurse must work in partnership with other professions and groups in public, private and voluntary sectors who have an impact on people's health and wellbeing. This book is written for new nurses whose placements may include working with children, adults, people with mental health issues and the community and who may in the future, work in many different contexts including health centres, primary care, walk-in centres, and specialist clinics such as Genitourinary Medicine and Sure Start areas as well as the acute hospital setting. Whilst specialist community public health nurses are recognised as making a specific contribution to the promotion of health and are registered on Part 3 of the Nursing and Midwifery Council (NMC) register, many other nurses have an interest in and responsibility for enabling people to achieve optimum health.

What is health promotion and public health?

Health promotion and public health have assumed increasing importance in nursing. In part this is a consequence of changing

1

understandings of medicine and health care. The World Health Report (2002) reports that ten risk factors account for about 40% of the 56 million deaths in the world each year and most of these can be addressed by public health measures such as tackling tobacco control or the nutrition of pregnant women. There is widespread recognition for the need to regulate the costs of, and control the demands for, health services. Preventing disease, for example, through infection-control measures, the modification of unhealthy lifestyles and the appropriate use of health services has been seen as offering a cheaper solution to demands for health care and threats to individual health.

The terms health promotion and public health are often used interchangeably. In this book we see these as complementary and overlapping areas of practice in which health promotion refers to efforts to prevent ill-health and promote positive health, a central aim being to enable people to take control over their own health. This may range from a relatively narrow focus on changing people's behaviour to community action or public policy change reflective of tackling the wider determinants of health. Public health has traditionally been associated with public health medicine and its efforts to prevent disease. It has been defined as 'the science and art of preventing disease, prolonging life and promoting health through the organised efforts of society' (Acheson, 1988). It takes a collective view of the health needs and health care of a population rather than an individual perspective. Its strategies thus include the assessment of the health of populations, formulating policies to prevent or manage health problems and significant disease conditions such as immunisation programmes and the promotion of healthy living environments and sustainable development.

Although health promotion and/or public health are central aspects of the nurse's job description, part of their training in the Common Foundation Programme and a core dimension in the NHS knowledge and skills framework for the competent nurse, these aspects of a nurse's role are not well understood. Health promotion is a difficult concept because there are many different perspectives on health which underpin current approaches. Many studies on perceptions of health find that it is a multidimensional concept which may co-exist with the presence of disease and in which people incorporate ideas about a positive sense of wellbeing and reserves of strength. For the nurse, promoting health means much more than the traditional role of addressing symptoms, experiences of pain, distress or discomfort. It means enabling people to increase control over their health, yet nursing is, according to Latter (2001), '. . . founded on a medical approach to care, characterised by an orientation towards cure, on treatment in the medical environment, a tendency to dismiss the patient's perspective and an expectation of the patient's role as one which involves passivity, trust and a willingness to wait for medical help'.

To promote health we need to understand how people learn, how messages are best communicated, how people make decisions about their health and how communities change. This means that we are drawing from many different disciplines – sociology, psychology, education and marketing to name but a few. However there is no discrete body of knowledge about public health or health promotion to be learned and for the nurse, this can be a source of frustration.

This book defines and illustrates what health promotion and public health mean in practice including their multidisciplinary nature and complex and wide ranging activities. It shows how nurses must look beyond traditional viewpoints: the biomedical mechanistic view of health in which patients present with a problem needing treatment and the expert-led approach to nursing in which patients are encouraged to adhere to advice. Instead, it suggests that a health promotion approach includes:

- a holistic view of health
- a focus on participatory approaches that involve patients in decision-making
- a focus on the determinants of health, the social, behavioural, economic and environmental conditions that are the root causes of health and illness which influence why patients now present for treatment or care
- multiple, complementary strategies to promote health at the individual and community level.

The three perspectives on health that influence health promotion practice are:

- the *biomedical* views health as the absence of diseases or disorders
- the *behavioural* views health as the product of making healthy lifestyle choices
- the *socio-environmental* views health as the product of social, economic and environmental determinants that provide incentives and barriers to the health of individuals and communities.

These perspectives represent three different ways of looking at health and influence the ways in which health issues are defined. They also influence the choice of strategies and actions for addressing health issues. If health is viewed simply as the absence of disease, then health promotion is seen as preventing disease principally through treatment and drug regimes. If health is viewed as the consequence of healthy lifestyles then health promotion is seen as education, communication of health messages, giving information and facilitating self help and mutual aid programmes. If, on the other hand, health is seen as a consequence of the socio-economic and environmental circumstances in which people live, then health promotion becomes a matter of tackling these issues to make healthy choices easier. The first two perspectives are much in evidence in nursing practice. A socio-economic and environmental perspective is more challenging for a setting which still emphasises one-to-one care.

Most hospital nurses have close and continuous contact with patients and at a time when they have a heightened awareness of their health (Latter, 2001). In the past, many nurses would employ a prescriptive approach to their practice, reassuring patients but intent on giving information usually about minor events such as the type of medication or a procedure. In order to be fulfilling their role, many felt they needed to be doing something **to** patients (Gott and O'Brien, 1990). Health promotion then was often characterised as 'nannying' due to the nurse assuming an expert role and telling patients what to do, ignoring the knowledge and experience that patients may already have about their own condition or lifestyle. Yet many nurses are taught that a basic principle underpinning practice should be to 'empower' patients. So what does it mean to foster empowerment? Empowerment in health promotion can be defined as a process through which people gain greater control over decisions and actions affecting their health (Nutbeam, 1998). To do this, the nurse needs to be able to clarify the individual's beliefs and values about health, health risks and health behaviours and help the patient to become aware of the factors that negatively and positively contribute to their health. Macleod Clark (1993) talked of this shift to 'well nursing' in which activities and interactions are characterised by participation – starting from the patient's health situation, to setting realistic goals and increasing their motivation and confidence, to taking action to improve their health. We see this as a health promoting way of working. But health promotion is far more than just developed interpersonal or counselling skills of active listening and open questioning.

Most of the guidance on modern nursing states that taking a public health/health promotion approach means:

- tackling the causes of ill health, not just responding to the consequences
- assessing the health needs of patients and developing programmes to address these needs rather than only responding to the needs of an individual
- planning work on the basis of local need, evidence and national health priorities rather than custom and practice.

Chapter overviews

This broad brief can make many nurses feel that health promotion is an activity concerning people in good health and therefore a concern for community nurses alone. Chapter 2 sets the scene by unpacking the concepts of health promotion and public health and exploring how these strategies have come to be at the centre of health care practice.

Chapter 3 summarises some of the evidence showing how social factors affect health. Inequalities in health status exist across geographical areas, social class, ethnicity and gender. People may also not have equal access to health services and often those most in need have least access or the worst services. The delivery of care may be discriminatory making it harder for individuals because of their language, race, age or disability. Material disadvantage has been shown to be a major factor not only directly in restricting opportunities for a healthy life but also indirectly in educational attainment and employment options. There is also emerging evidence of psychosocial risk factors for poor health especially weak social networks and stress in early life.

Current health policy is committed to tackling inequalities in health and a raft of government legislation is designed to: address areas of deprivation, increase the opportunities for disadvantaged and marginalised groups and take children out of poverty. However, much health policy is characterised by a focus on individual responsibility – the recent Government White Paper on public health is, for example, entitled *Choosing Health: making healthy choices easier* (DoH, 2004). Public health thus reflects ideological debates about the rights and responsibilities of individuals and the state for the nation's health. Throughout this book we challenge the individualistic model which focuses on the presenting patient's problems alone and encourage the nurse to be aware of significant economic or social circumstances that might make it difficult for individuals, families and communities to adopt or experience healthier lifestyles despite being informed and offered advice. We urge the nurse to avoid victim blaming in which individuals are encouraged to feel responsible and guilty for their own health status. This sort of approach runs the risk of increasing inequalities by which only the most educated, articulate and confident individuals will be able to accept and adopt health messages.

Chapter 4 discusses the various models of health promotion which have attempted to describe approaches to a health issue. Many practitioners do not use theory when planning health promotion and work far more from intuition or existing practice wisdom which is often rooted in a traditional health education approach. Health promotion models are not, by and large, planning models but attempts to 'scope' the broad field of health promotion. Beattie's typology (1991) for example, illustrates how health promotion activities may take place at an individual or collective level. They may be expert-led (authoritative) or undertaken in partnership with clients (negotiated). Nevertheless an awareness of health promotion models and models of behaviour change encourages much more rigour in planning, making the practitioner be explicit about what they are trying to do and articulating those determinants that are thought to influence behavioural or clinical outcomes and which they think can be changed. An effective project or intervention, even if it is simply a one to one education session, will benefit from explicitly stated goals, methods and means of evaluation showing how any change following the intervention can be demonstrated.

Policy is an integral part of nursing yet there is an assumption about policies developed at the organisational level to provide more effective and efficient services and at a national and local level to improve health. Health promotion is an inherently political activity, reflecting current ideologies about the organisation of society and the extent to which people are connected to each other, society's health and social care provision, the extent of personal responsibility, legitimate means to encourage choice and the role of government legislation (Naidoo and Wills, 2000). An understanding of the national and local policy agenda will help the nurse identify how they can make an explicit contribution to meeting targets and priorities for health improvement (e.g. childhood obesity, sexual health, accidents and substance misuse). Policy analysis helps the practitioner 'to understand the multiple and sometimes conflicting facets of the policy process that contribute to multiple outcomes – some intended and some unintended' and their own role in implementation (Walt, 1994). Chapter 5 discusses current public health priorities and some of the many targets set by the government aimed at improving the health of the population. These are contained in a number of policy documents:

- The NHS Plan: a plan for investment, a plan for reform (DoH, 2000)
- National Service Frameworks offer detailed guidance about standards of services for older people, children, mental health, diabetes, coronary heart disease (CHD), cancer and long-term conditions
- The White Paper *Choosing Health* sets out a wide range of proposed actions to address major public health problems.

These priorities need to be considered in conjunction with a number of national targets that have been set over the past few years. In 1998, Saving Lives: Our Healthier Nation (DoH, 1998) listed targets aimed at reducing deaths from the four main killers: cancer, CHD and stroke, accidents and mental illness. This was followed in 2001 by two national inequalities targets, one relating to infant mortality and the other to life expectancy:

- starting with children under one year, by 2010 to reduce by at least 10% the gap in mortality between manual groups and the population as a whole
- starting with Health Authorities, by 2010 to reduce by at least 10% the gap between the fifth of areas with the lowest life expectancy at birth and the population as a whole.

The chapter discusses why certain health issues become national priorities, why the nurse should be involved and some examples of actions they can take as advocates for local public health initiatives.

Whilst nurses may see practice as focusing on individuals and families, many recognise the need for a wider understanding of the health of local populations or communities and a service directed towards those with greatest needs. Using existing information to identify the main issues, the contributory factors and who is affected will help identify the most appropriate interventions. Last (2001) describes epidemiology as 'completing the clinical picture', with its methods therefore being an important tool of nursing practice in helping to plan and determine health policy. Despite this, according to Whitehead (2000) it seems to be poorly understood and greatly underused by the nursing profession. Chapter 6 outlines some of the key concepts associated with using existing data sources to describe a population's health. As a lone practitioner or with others, the nurse may need to gather and generate data from a variety of sources to assess health needs and then to agree priorities for action and local health plans. This information will also help influence resource allocation to areas of greatest health and social need. For example, the School Nurse Practice Development Resource Pack (2006) describes a core competency for school nurses to 'Work with children, young people, parents/carers and colleagues from other sectors to assess the needs of a school population and develop a school health plan'.

The next three chapters in the book, Chapters 7–9, discuss the key strategies involved in promoting health: infection control and health protection; promoting healthy lifestyles through behavioural change; working in and with communities and how nurses can seek to engage and involve local populations.

Disease surveillance, particularly of communicable disease, is a core public health function and Chapter 7 outlines the principles of screening and vaccination programmes. A major hazard associated with hospital admission is the risk of acquiring an infection. Whilst the challenge of monitoring, controlling and treating methicillin-resistant *Staphylococcus aureus* (MRSA) may lie with a specialist infection control nurse, all health professionals in secondary care are responsible for the basic aspect of their role – hygiene. Hand washing is the single most important action a nurse can take which can reduce the spread of disease. Chapter 7 also discusses the key role for the nurse in communicating about risk. Sometimes a nurse wishes to convey to a patient the risk associated with their behaviour or they may wish to discuss the risks associated with a particular intervention. Increasingly, understanding the role of gene mutations has led to the development of targeted risk management and preventative strategies. For example, familial breast cancer clinics have been set up to address the needs of women concerned about their perceived risk of developing breast cancer because they have a relative with the disease.

Chapter 8 focuses on the promotion of healthy lifestyles. 50% of cardiovascular diseases among those above the age of 30 years can be attributed to suboptimal blood pressure, 31% to high cholesterol and 14% to tobacco, yet the estimated joint effects of these three risks amount to about 65% of cardiovascular diseases in this group (World Health Report, 2002). Nutrition, smoking and physical activity behaviours are then key to reducing CHD. There are numerous opportunities for the nurse to encourage behaviour change and underpinning such an approach are the objectives of increasing awareness of health information, developing self efficacy through better decision making, assertiveness and interpersonal skills. The lifestyle perspective is however, an individualistic one in which people are encouraged to change health behaviours irrespective of their power to do so. The social, environmental and economic conditions that make the adoption of health choices easier should not be ignored and encouraging individuals to think about their lives and the factors determining their health is part of what the Tones and Tilford (2001) model of health promotion calls critical consciousness raising.

The methods, values and philosophy of community development offer a way of addressing population health by putting 'community' at the centre. Chapter 9 shows how it demands a strategic approach that addresses the social conditions that create poor health and develops the services and programmes needed by communities. Community development methods support and help the public to identify what they need. It offers a challenge for nurses because it means working **with** the public and client groups not for them. When these principles are applied to the hospital setting, they encourage nurses to be more participatory, involving patients in decision making and care planning. Developing the capacity and confidence of individuals, groups, families and communities to influence and use services and take control over the factors influencing their health, be these informational, behavioural or environmental factors, is at the heart of health promotion work.

The task-oriented culture of hospitals and little time for extended patient contact means health promotion is often a peripheral activity, even though episodes of acute illness or injury can be seen as windows of opportunity for advice and education on disease self-management, rehabilitation and to empower patients to make better use of health services. The final chapter, Chapter 10, discusses how the hospital can be a more health promoting setting. As the hospital is part of the community, so creating supportive environments for health means integrating the hospital with wider health concerns such as sustainable development and environmental management. Within the hospital itself, promoting health would mean closer relationships of different disciplines such as occupational health, infection control, catering managers and new structures for patient and public involvement. The chapter describes the World Health Organization Health Promoting Hospital movement and its call for hospitals to be at the heart of their communities and part of a seamless service that addresses health services across the whole health and social care continuum. The modern nurse, whatever their context, recognises that they work in partnership with others in a multi-agency, multi-professional team to improve health and wellbeing.

Conclusion

There are few examples of effective health promotion in nursing practice (Schickler *et al*, 2002) and so it is often taken as simply meaning to offer advice on leading a healthy lifestyle and is thus interpreted as an add-on activity to a busy and care-oriented job. Despite this, UK national governing bodies such as the Royal College of Nursing and the Nursing and Midwifery Council have encouraged nurses to take a more health-promoting role. As Whitehead (2005) states for the most part, nursing 'has failed to seize upon their opportunity and at best, only paid lip service to the presented opportunities. Nurses have remained firmly entrenched within the ritualised and traditional functions of limited and limiting health education practices'. Why is this? Throughout this book we have presented the opportunities that exist for the nurse to promote health and the knowledge, skills and attitudes necessary to do so. No apology is made for rooting these in a biomedical framework since this is how most nurses work. However, the intention of this book is also to encourage a different mind-set with a much broader agenda which acknowledges the socio-political determinants of health and the necessity of the nurse contributing to the creation of supportive environments within a healthy public policy framework. In summary, there are several themes that run through this book:

- *Health* rather than health care, in particular the social and environmental influences on health and how these need to be addressed to improve health.
- *Social justice* which involves tackling inequalities in health, in particular poverty and social inclusion of individuals, families and communities.
- *Participation* in service development and delivery so patients and users are empowered to take responsibility for their own health.
- *Collaboration and partnership* between professionals, private, public and voluntary sectors and across agencies.
- *Information, research and evidence* to provide a sound base for practice.

References

Acheson D. (1988) *Public Health in England: report of the committee of inquiry into the future development of the public health function.* London, HMSO.

Beattie A. (1991) Knowledge and control in health promotion: a test case for social policy and social theory. In Gabe J. Calnan M. and Bury M. (Eds.) *The Sociology of the Health Service.* London, Routledge.

Department of Health (1998) *Saving Lives: Our Healthier Nation.* The Stationery Office, London.

Department of Health (2000) *The NHS Plan: a plan for investment, a plan for reform.* DoH, London.

Department of Health (2004) *Choosing Health: making healthier choices easier.* DoH, London.

Department of Health (2006) *School Nurse: Practice Development Resource Pack.* DoH, London.

Gott M. and O'Brien M. (1990) The role of the nurse in health promotion, *Health Promotion International*, **5**, 2, 137–43.

Last J. (2001) *A dictionary of epidemiology* 4th ed. Oxford, Oxford University Press.

Latter S. (2001) The potential for health promotion in hospital nursing practice. In Scriven A. and Orme J. (Eds.) *Health Promotion: Professional Perspectives* (p 75). Basingstoke, Palgrave Macmillan.

MacLeod Clark S. (1993) From sick nursing to well nursing: evolution or revolution? In Wilson Barnett J. and Macleod Clark J. (Eds.) *Research in Health Promotion and Nursing.* Basingstoke, Palgrave Macmillan.

Naidoo J. and Wills J. (2000) *Health Promotion: Foundations for Practice* 2nd ed. London, Ballière Tindall.

Nutbeam D. (1998) Health Promotion Glossary, *Health Promotion International*, **13**, 349–64.

Schickler P. James T. and Smith P. (2002) How do I know it's health promotion? A study of health promotion activities and awareness in student placements, *Learning in Health and Social Care*, **1**, 4, 218–28.

Tones K. and Tilford S. (2001) *Health promotion: effectiveness, efficiency and equity* 3rd ed. Cheltenham, Nelson Thornes.

Walt G. (1994) *Health Policy: An Introduction to Process and Power* (p 40). London, Zed Books Ltd.

Whitehead D. (2000) Is there a place for epidemiology in Nursing?, *Nursing Standard*, **14**, 42, 35–9.

Whitehead D. (2005) The culture, context and progress of health promotion in nursing. In Scriven A. (Ed.) *Health Promoting Practice: the contribution of nurses and allied health professionals* (p 19). Basingstoke, Palgrave Macmillan.

World Health Organization (2002) *World Health Report 2002–reducing risks, promoting healthy life.* WHO, Geneva.

Health and Health Promotion

Linda Jackson

Introduction

This chapter considers the concept of health and why it is central to the practice of all health care professionals. There are many ways that the concept of health can be understood. The traditional medical model, where health is seen as the absence of disease and illness, has led to the perception that health is an individual phenomenon for which each person is responsible. This chapter will encourage nurses to explore other concepts of health including a social model of health that focuses on the social and political determinants of health and the unequal access that people may have to opportunities to improve their health. This chapter will look at the definitions for health promotion and public health. As these are basic and commonly used terms, it is important to clearly define and examine what is meant by them and how they are applied to nursing practice. By exploring other concepts of health it will challenge nursing students to consider whether, in addition to the more reactive nursing role of responding to disease and illness, they also have a proactive role in promoting health.

Learning outcomes

By the end of this chapter you will be able to:

- analyse the difference between a medical and social model of health
- discuss health promotion and apply it to nursing practice
- define and discuss the concepts of public health and 'new public health' and how they apply to nursing practice.

Definitions of health and wellbeing

Health can be hard to define, as it is one of those words that can mean many different things to different people. It is often looked at in two main ways:

- a positive or wellness approach where health is viewed as an asset or the ability to do something
- a more negative approach which focuses on the absence of illness and diseases.

This medical model of health sees health as being about illness and disease and ill health determined by the individual patient or person. It has been challenged as being an inadequate way of explaining the complexities of health and illness. Even with adequate medical treatment and access to health services many people still suffer from ill health. A social model of health sees health as involving all of society not just the individual person (Dahlgren and Whitehead, 1991).

Activity

Would you describe yourself as healthy or unhealthy? Write down a list of factors, e.g. personal, medical, internal or external, which you think have a bearing on your health.

Some of the factors that you came up with might have been genetic makeup, family, culture, religion, friends, lifestyle, health services, housing, employment status, self-esteem and many more. The World Health Organization (WHO) defined health as a 'state of complete physical, mental and social well-being and not merely the absence of disease or infirmity' (WHO, 1948). In addition to addressing health in a positive sense, it is noteworthy that mental health was stressed as well as physical and social aspects of health and individual wellbeing. This can be seen as a more 'holistic' approach to health.

Activity

In nursing practice what are the advantages of using the WHO definition of health?

The WHO definition takes in the whole person and looks beyond their physical health. It acknowledges that a person may have a profound sense of health and wellbeing even though they may have a disease and conversely, that a person is not necessarily healthy just because there is no diagnosable pathology.

There has been a growing recognition that people may not see health or define it in the same way as health professionals. Three main findings related to the definition of health have been identified in research:

- health is not being ill
- it is a necessary prerequisite for life's functions
- it is a sense of wellbeing expressed in physical and mental terms (Blaxter, 1990).

The WHO's more positive definition of health reflects more accurately how ordinary people view their health than the more medical perspective. Health is viewed differently at different times of life and by the different genders. It is also a dynamic state where each person's potential is different and each person's health needs are different.

Scenario

Consider the following patients and their concept of health.

One is a middle-aged patient living with a chronic condition, e.g. human immunodeficiency virus (HIV). The other is an older patient with limited mobility who lives alone.

What might their concept of health be and how might it be different to that of the nurse?

The patient living with HIV might consider himself healthy if he is able to work and do the things he enjoys in life. His major concern might be looking healthy enough so no one knows that he has a chronic condition which might affect his long-term work prospects as work for him might not only offer a financial reward but also a social support network. It would be important to first ask the patient how he is coping and what he considers to be the most important aspect of living with the disease as opposed to focusing on monitoring physical signs and symptoms and getting blood work done.

For the older patient with limited mobility, health is more than restoration of mobility – it is improving quality of life. His major concern may be depression, social isolation and anxiety which all impact on his health and wellbeing. The health promotion role could involve listening to the patient and trying to identify his needs as he sees them and offering emotional support. The nurse might take more of a functional view of the patient's health and may focus on his ability to perform selected duties of everyday life, e.g., dressing, cooking, climbing stairs and moving about unaided. The patient's mental health may or may not be assessed, however, this may be the most important issue for this patient.

Influences on health

As previously mentioned, there are many factors other than lifestyle that influence or determine a person's health. These include (Acheson, 1998):

- living conditions
- employment (or unemployment)
- education
- occupation
- income
- social networks
- access to health services and care
- family history.

These influences are well illustrated in the model by Dahlgren and Whitehead (1991) presented in Figure 2.1. It clearly shows the difference between individual and social factors, with an onion likeness, whereby each layer can be peeled away. The core consists of inherited factors that are fixed. The inner layer suggests that health is partly determined by lifestyle factors such as smoking, physical activity and diet. Moving outwards the diagram draws attention to relationships with family, friends and others in the community. The next layer focuses on living and working conditions – housing, employment, income, access to services and education among other factors. The outer layer shows the

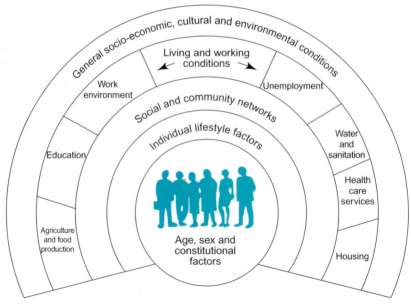

Figure 2.1 Influences on health. Reproduced with permission from Dahlgren and Whitehead (1991), Policies and strategies to promote social equity in health, Stockholm Institute for Future Studies.

overarching umbrella of the broader socio-economic, cultural and environmental conditions that affect health. This also includes political change, social forces and structures. It can be seen from this that the issues that impact on health are complex and much wider than individual lifestyle choices.

Many things affect our health – what we have to eat, where we work, where we live, the air we breathe, the germs we come in contact with and our genes. Housing might not be the first thing to come to mind when thinking about health, however, it is of particular importance to health with increased risks of asthma and even coronary heart disease (CHD) associated with poor housing. Before reading the evidence below, consider the following questions:

- Why is housing relevant to health (specifically CHD)?
- What might the evidence be of the impact of housing on health?
- If it is relevant, what action or intervention might be needed and who will benefit from it?
- What would be the key targets?

Case study 2.1: Housing and CHD

Why is housing relevant to health?
When room temperatures fall below 12°C cardiovascular changes can be seen that increase the risk of myocardial infarction and stroke.

Impact of housing on health?
There is excess mortality in Britain in the winter. Approximately 40 000 more people die in Britain in winter than in summer and most of these are older people. These excess deaths are mostly due to respiratory and cardiovascular diseases, not hypothermia. Therefore the risk to health increases as temperature decreases.

What action/intervention is needed?
Standards need to be set so that an acceptable indoor temperature, e.g. 20°C, can be achieved at no more than 10% of the household income. Any excess should be paid for in social benefits.

Who will benefit?
The poorest in society: the unemployed, the chronically ill, older people. 'Fuel poverty' describes those with least to spend on heating but living in houses that are hard to heat. Many low cost houses are prone to damp and cold.

What are the key targets?
Indoor temperature of local authority housing stock to be kept to a minimum of 20°C.

Source: Hicks and Crowther (2000)

Many people trained in a medical model of health find it difficult to think about a chronic health condition like CHD in terms of the social and environmental factors that impact on the condition. This example may suggest some new ways of considering what influences people's health. There are further readings mentioned at the end of this chapter on the social model of health and the wider influences on health.

Health education and health promotion

Health education and health promotion are often thought to mean the same thing, however, they are not. Simply put, 'health education is part of, but not the sum of, health promotion' (Gott and O'Brien, 1990). Education is one of the means of improving health and is often the main one that is used by health professionals. Health education is concerned with communicating information and with building the motivation, skills and confidence necessary to take action to improve health (see Chapter 8).

Part of the nursing role is to promote the health of patients and clients and this is often done through education. This can take place at three different levels. However, because nurses mostly work with patients who are already ill, the emphasis has mostly been on secondary or tertiary prevention:

- Primary prevention – strategies to reduce the risk of onset of ill-health, e.g., immunisation.
- Secondary prevention – seeks to shorten episodes of illness and prevent the secondary progression of ill-health through early diagnosis and treatment, e.g., screening.
- Tertiary prevention – seeks to limit the disability or complications arising from an irreversible condition, such as controlling pain or through rehabilitation after a heart attack (Naidoo and Wills, 2000).

> **Activity**
>
> Can you think of specific examples of primary, secondary and tertiary prevention that nurses can do in relation to CHD?

The following are all examples of preventative activities relating to CHD (DoH, 1999):

- Nurse-led blood pressure clinics to identify and help manage hypo/hypertension and medication compliance (secondary)
- Smoking cessation clinics using national smoking cessation guidelines (secondary)

- 'Healthy lifestyle' clinics in collaboration with other health professionals to address factors such as diet, nutrition and exercise (primary)
- Cholesterol clinics to assist in risk factor identification and management (secondary)
- Care for patients with congestive cardiac failure under home-based initiatives (tertiary)
- Nurse-led chest pain clinics or risk factor screening and reduction clinics (secondary)
- The coordination and delivery of cardiac rehabilitation programmes in conjunction with other health care professionals (tertiary).

As you can see from the examples of preventative activities relating to CHD, most nursing interventions are not primary interventions. Health promotion, on the other hand, is about improving the health status of individuals and communities. It is a broader term that can be visualised like an umbrella that has, education, as well as, social, environmental, political and economic components under its cover to improve and promote health (Nutbeam, 1998). Often the word 'promotion' when used in the context of health promotion is associated with the idea of media and even propaganda. This is a misunderstanding of the term. Promotion, in this context, is about improving health at all levels from individuals to society to worldwide policy and supporting and encouraging it to be higher on personal and public agendas.

As discussed earlier, the factors that determine a person's health are often outside their control. Therefore, a fundamental aspect of health promotion is that it aims to empower people to have more control over aspects of their lives that affect their health. A landmark international WHO conference on health promotion was held in Ottawa Canada in 1986 and it published the key document the *Ottawa Charter for Health Promotion*, which continues to guide health promotion practice today. 'Health promotion is the process of enabling people to increase control over and to improve their health.' (WHO, 1986): this definition combines these two elements of improving health and having more control over it.

The Ottawa Charter provides five action areas that are central to the conceptual framework of health promotion:

- build healthy public policy
- create supportive environments
- develop personal skills
- reorient health services
- strengthen community action (WHO, 1986; Nutbeam, 1998).

These five areas suggest that for the health of the population to be improved, it is important not only to help individuals to lead healthier lives but to make it easier for them to do so, e.g. encouraging healthy

Table 2.1 Ottawa Charter.

Ottawa Charter Action Areas	Examples
Build healthy public policy	• No smoking policy in public buildings including all National Health Service (NHS) buildings • Breastfeeding policy in hospitals • Motorcycle helmet laws • Drink driving policies and laws
Create supportive environments	• Healthy food choices for staff in workplaces (including hospital canteens) • Healthy school meals for children • Easy access to condoms (including reasonable prices) • Safe and well lit play and walking areas
Develop personal skills	• Smoking cessation skills • Information on health issues • Food product label reading • Parenting skills
Reorient health services	• Blood pressure screening at chemists • Breastfeeding support services in the community • Immunisation clinics at neighbourhood clinics or surgeries • Chlamydia screening on mobile buses in areas where young people can access them

workplaces (see Chapter 10) and supporting a physical environment that is more conducive to health with 'green' public transport and locally grown fresh food. Other examples of these action areas are listed in Table 2.1. Can you think of any others?

The health promotion role of most nurses will be in developing personal skills for their clients and patients (see Chapter 8). The aim of these activities is to help people feel more confident and competent in:

• accessing and use of the health care system
• assessing their own risks to health and decision-making about their health lifestyle
• understanding the economic, social and environmental influences on their health.

In order to demonstrate how health promotion can be integrated into nursing practice, the next section will discuss two scenarios of nurses in acute and community settings. In each scenario, consider the following questions:

- What would be the likely health needs of the patient?
- What is the health promotion role of the nurse?
- Are the patient and the nurse likely to share the same perspective on health?
- What else, if anything, could the nurse do to promote the health of the patient/client?

Scenario

Patient on a ward with a myocardial infarction (MI).

Patient priorities are likely to be to resume daily activities and be able to go home quickly. This may be the nurse's concern as well but may not be the nurse's priority. The nurse's health promotion role would include: listening to patient's concerns and needs – not just giving information; involving the patient/client in their health care plan; providing information and skills to decrease heart disease risk factors; awareness of patient's living situation when returning home (e.g., cooking facilities, transport, support in the home); referral information to community programmes on patient's needs (e.g., smoking, walking, cooking). The nurse may also prioritise health education advice and behaviour change e.g. smoking, activity and diet.

Scenario

Young mother with a three month old baby attends a mother and baby clinic held at her local community centre every week. The health visitor not only checks the baby's progress but asks the mother how she is coping and allows time for her to talk. Other mothers attend the clinic at the same time and they wait in the same area and compare stories.

The priorities of the client here will be wider than just the developmental progress of the baby. For a new mother, health may be a very wide concept, including every aspect of her life, including her sexual, emotional, mental and physical wellbeing. It would also include her relationship with her partner and his support.

The health promotion role of the nurse would include:

- establishing the client's priorities
- monitoring the progress of the baby
- acting as a source of information
- listening and talking (finding out how the client is coping by asking her how she is)
- building up coping skills

Continued

- acting as a referral to other agencies
- initiating a social support network (of new mothers attending the clinic)

In this case, nurse and client are likely to share a similar perspective. Often, the focus of much antenatal and postnatal care is on the early identification of health problems, instead of the development of the coping skills of the mother. Working with individuals should be based on a partnership that focuses on identifying the issues the family would like to address and helping them to express their needs and choices. For the practitioner this may involve understanding a view of health that is different from their own and allowing enough time for the conversation to evolve.

The practitioner may see a broader public health role in looking at the factors contributing to the client's role as a new mother, such as social isolation, parenting anxiety and gender roles.

The role of social support is increasingly being recognised as crucial in the maintenance of positive health.

Public health and the new public health

It has been said that some people need health care some of the time but all people need public health all of the time. This notion of public health demonstrates the prominent role that public health has played in society in the last century and a half. Dramatic improvements were made to the public's health in the mid nineteenth century. Early pioneers recognised that poor health, for much of the population, came from poverty and dreadful living conditions. The types of action taken to improve health included legislation and regulations to tackle:

- housing standards, e.g. 1855 Nuisance Removal Act; 1875 Artisan Dwelling Act
- sanitation and clean water, e.g. 1866 Sanitary Act
- regulation of food, e.g. 1848 Public Health Act
- regulation of workplaces, e.g. 1864 Factory Act.

Mortality declined in the late nineteenth century, largely due to rising living standards and this expansion of preventive public health measures. Following this the introduction of vaccines and antibiotics in the post World War II period also had a positive impact on health status and mortality. This started to move the focus away from population health to more personal medical services. In the 1950s and 60s the focus shifted towards the need for changes in individual health behaviour about issues such as sexually transmitted infections, family planning, weight control, alcohol consumption and smoking and a corresponding emphasis on health education. During the 1970s this focus was criticised because it moved the attention away from the social and economic determinants of health and tended to blame individuals for their own ill-health. This was known as 'victim blaming' and it still happens today.

In the 1980s the pendulum swung again and there emerged the broader approach of health promotion and public health we see now. It was called the 'new public health'. It includes health education but also political and social action to address issues such as employment, discrimination, poverty and the environment where people live. It also focuses on the grass roots involvement of people in their communities shaping their future. The goals of the 'new public health' are closely aligned with those of the World Health Organization in their 'Health for All by the Year 2000' initiative (WHO, 1981). This new public health initiative offers a strategy that works towards developing healthy public policies, working with communities to identify their own needs and building a more enabling health care system with a focus on prevention. It is underpinned by:

- intersectoral collaboration (or partnership working)
- community participation
- equity.

A more formal and current definition of public health is: 'the science and art of preventing disease, prolonging life and promoting health through organised efforts of society' (Acheson, 1988). A similar definition is offered for public health in nursing: '*Public health in nursing, midwifery and health visiting practice is about commissioning health services and providing professional care through organised collaboration in the NHS and society, to protect and promote health and well-being, prolong life and prevent ill-health in local communities and groups and populations*' (Craig and Lindsay, 2000).

Through this definition it can be seen that nurses are viewed as having a role in preventing harm and providing protection to communities. Public health goes beyond what has traditionally been described as good nursing practice. It focuses on understanding the social and economic causes of health and ill-health and is concerned with interventions at the community or social, as well as individual level. When working with individual patients, it is important to understand what has brought them to you in the first place. This is illustrated in the story by McKinlay (Box 2.1).

As Naidoo and Wills (2000) point out, the concept of refocusing upstream is a powerful and persuasive argument for health promotion. It can help us to change our thinking from the belief that medical care can, or will, solve most help problems towards thinking about prevention.

> **Box 2.1** A story about prevention and persuading us to refocus 'upstream' (McKinlay, 1979)
>
> There I am standing by the shore of a swiftly flowing river and I hear the cry of a drowning man. So I jump into the river, put my arms around him, pull him to shore and apply artificial respiration. Just when he begins to breathe, there is another cry for help. So I jump into the river, reach him, pull him to shore, apply artificial respiration, and just as he begins to breathe, another cry for help. So back into the river again, reaching, pulling, applying, breathing and then another yell. Again and again goes the sequence. You know I am so busy jumping in, pulling them to shore, applying artificial respiration, that I have no time to see who the hell is upstream pushing them all in.

The nurse's role in promoting health

Health promotion is increasingly important to nursing practice. It enhances the way in which health care and services are viewed, looking beyond the medical model to consider the broader influences on health. It can be seen from previous discussions in this chapter that health promotion shares many of the characteristics of good nursing practice:

- it is client-centred: it is based on an assessment of the client's individual needs and valuing the client's own views
- it includes spending time listening and talking to client's individual needs and using high level communication skills and methods
- it seeks to involve clients in their own health care decisions.

Gott and O'Brien (1990) in their study on the role of the nurse in health promotion, reported that generally nurses seemed enthusiastic about health promotion and considered themselves to have a role to play. However, that role was not as well defined or as certain as stated. They report that although health promotion is being taught in the nursing curriculum it has tended to focus on communication and therefore health education along with the principles of health promotion practice: empowerment, equity, collaboration, participation. Many nurses reported that they felt health promotion was part of their work but they were unsure how to do it. A challenge remains for how to integrate and apply these principles to nursing practice. For many nurses, health promotion work might be short-term or individually driven. This will be particularly true for hospital nurses. Community nurses (especially health visitors and community midwives) have more opportunities for family and community intervention.

In terms of public health, the Standing Nursing and Midwifery Advisory Committee (SNMAC) published a report in 1995 outlining the role nurses should play in public health. It was entitled *Making it Happen* and it suggested that while some nurses, such as health visitors, school nurses, occupational health nurses and those working with communicable disease were already doing public health work, there was scope for many others to increase their contribution to public health to the benefit of patients. The report encourages nurses in every type of practice to become 'thoughtful in promoting public health strategies and interventions, working together with the people and communities they serve' (SNMAC, 1995). The types of public health work that nurses traditionally do include:

- infection control
- screening
- carrying out immunisation programmes.

Other nursing contributions could include:

- health profiling
- community development approaches to meeting need
- working in partnerships to provide more relevant services.

Case study 2.2 illustrates how primary care nurses can extend their role beyond the practice setting and treatment orientation to start looking upstream to see how they can prevent accidents from happening in the first place.

Case study 2.2: Public health in primary care – preventing accidents in young children

After reviewing the Primary Care Trust (PCT) annual report and caseload reports, a primary care team was concerned about the number of accidents in young children. However, they did not have a true picture of what was happening. The team worked in an area with high levels of deprivation and they were aware that the children most likely to suffer from accidents were from low-income families. Discussions with the general practitioners (GPs) and health visitors indicated that this was true. They were also aware that accident prevention was one of the Government's key targets for health improvement so it seemed reasonable to include accidents as one of their three main priorities for the coming year. Their action plan had several components:

Continued

(1) *Keep better statistics within the practice.* This meant agreeing on terminology, e.g. definition of children. They agreed a definition of all youngsters under the age of 14. In order to have accurate data, they had to design a computer code for recording accidents that could be used by everyone. To obtain more complete data they linked with the paediatric liaison health visitor at Accident and Emergency (A&E) who agreed to encourage parents to record accidents that need home treatment in the parent-held record.

(2) *Raise awareness in the community.* To raise awareness of accidents locally, information was posted on the notice boards at the local health centre and members of the team visited 'mothers and toddlers groups' to talk about local accidents. In addition they mapped out accident danger zones to present to the local council. First aid classes were offered to parents in the schools, which were advertised in the school newsletter.

(3) *Ensuring a safer environment.* They built partnerships with schools, local agencies, Sure Start programmes and housing estates to develop safe play areas for children and to set up a safety equipment loan scheme for such items as fire, stair and cooker guards. In addition, they contacted the local fire brigade who were keen to extend the use of smoke detectors in homes and to talk to people about how to use them successfully.

(4) *Improved treatment.* All staff in primary care were offered instruction in first aid treatment.

(5) *Evaluation.* The evaluation was set up at the beginning of the programme. It included:
- audit of the completeness of the accident data on the practice computer at year end
- audit of all childhood accidents to highlight trends
- audit of the resources for home safety that had been supplied to determine the percentage of households that had safety equipment
- process evaluation at the end of the first aid sessions
- production of a joint accident prevention plan with all local agencies.

Source: Morgan (2000)

Summary

This chapter has considered definitions and concepts in order to set the stage for the rest of the book. It has defined the medical and social models of health and encouraged health practitioners to look beyond the medical model to consider the broader social and environmental determinants of health. The origins of health promotion were discussed and there was a discussion of the difference between health promotion and health education. Health promotion is a broad concept encompassing health education but not the same thing. People working in health promotion need to have a clear understanding of health, the aspect of health that is being promoted and the ways in which health is determined by wider influences than individual behaviour. In addition, this chapter covered the history of public health and how the 'new public health' has built upon those early nineteenth century public health concerns. The new public health includes more of the social determinants of health and draws on a larger group of partners, including policy makers, environmental health workers and international agencies. The application of health promotion and public health work to nursing practice has been illustrated through numerous case studies and scenarios.

Further reading and resources

Department of Health (2004) *Choosing Health: making healthier choices easier.* London, DoH.

This White Paper sets out the key principles for supporting the public to make healthier and more informed choices with regard to health. It is followed by delivery and action plans which can be found on the same website. http://www.dh.gov.uk/PublicationsAndStatistics/Publications/PublicationsPolicy AndGuidance/

Ewles L. and Simnett I. (2003) *Promoting Health: A Practical Guide* 5th ed. London, Ballière Tindall.

This text is a popular basic text on health promotion and provides comprehensive and readable information on the theory and practice of health promotion. It includes questionnaires, practical exercises and case studies.

Naidoo J. and Wills J. (2000) *Health Promotion: Foundations for Practice* 2nd ed. London, Ballière Tindall.

This wide-ranging text provides a comprehensive and critical framework for promoting health. There are in-depth discussions, reflection points and case studies. It is reader-centred and an excellent resource for anyone interested in this field.

World Health Organization (1986) *Ottawa Charter for Health Promotion.* WHO, Copenhagen.

The first International Conference on Health Promotion met in Ottawa, Canada on the 21 November 1986 and developed this Charter for action to achieve health for all by the year 2000 and beyond. This conference was primarily a response to growing expectations for a new public health movement around the world. Discussions focused on the needs in industrialised countries, but took into account similar concerns in all other regions. It built on the progress made through the 'Declaration on Primary Health Care' at Alma-Ata, the World Health Organization's 'Targets for Health for All' document, and the recent debate at the World Health Assembly on intersectoral action for health. The Charter is still widely used today as a framework for action in health promotion.
http://www.who.int/healthpromotion/conferences/previous/ottawa/en/

World Health Organization (1999) *Health 21: the health for all policy framework for WHO European region.* WHO, Copenhagen.

The WHO European programmes features the need to understand the wider social influences on health and this text brings the latest targets for public health and health promotion up to date in a very readable format.

References

Acheson D. (1988) *Public Health in England. report of the committee of inquiry into the future of the public health function.* London, HMSO.

Acheson D. (1998) *Independent Inquiry into Inequalities and Health.* London, The Stationery Office.

Blaxter M. (1990) *Health and Lifestyle.* London, Routledge.

Craig P. and Lindsay G. (2000) *Nursing for Public Health: population based care* (p 130). London, Churchill Livingstone.

Dahlgren G. and Whitehead M. (1991) *Policies and strategies to promote social equity in health.* Stockholm, Institute for Future Studies.

Department of Health (1999) *Making a difference: strengthening the nursing, midwifery and health visiting contribution to health and healthcare.* DoH, London.

Gott M. and O'Brien M. (1990) The role of the nurse in health promotion, *Health Promotion International,* **5**, 2, 137–43.

Hicks NR. and Crowther R. (2000) Coronary heart disease: a practical tool and structured approach to developing and implementing a HimP. In Rawaf S. and Orton P. *Health improvement programmes.* London, Royal Society of Medicine.

McKinlay JB. (1979) A case for refocusing upstream: the political economy of sickness. In Jaco EG. (Ed.) *Patients, Physicians, and Illness: A Sourcebook in Behavioural Science and Health*. New York, Free Press.

Morgan M. (2000) Public Health – What does it mean for nurses in primary care? In Carey L. (Ed.) *Practice Nursing*. London, Ballière Tindall.

Naidoo J. and Wills J. (2000) *Health Promotion: Foundations for Practice* 2nd ed. London, Ballière Tindall.

Nutbeam D. (1998) Health Promotion Glossary, *Health Promotion International*, **13**, 349–64.

Standing Nursing and Midwifery Advisory Committee (SNMAC) (1995) *Making it Happen*. HMSO, London.

World Health Organization (1948) *Constitution*. WHO, Geneva.

World Health Organization (1981) *Regional strategy for attaining Health for All by the year 2000*. WHO, Copenhagen.

World Health Organization (1986) *Ottawa Charter for Health Promotion*. WHO, Geneva.

3

Influences on Health

Jenny Husbands

Introduction

Health and disease are determined by factors in the wider socio-economic and physical environment. Low income and inadequate housing for example, may limit people's ability to take control or have any power to alter the conditions affecting their health. Understanding those factors that impact on a patient's health and their capacity to develop and maintain good health is a vital aspect of the nurse's role.

Although health status is improving in the UK with people living longer and early mortality from many diseases declining, these improvements have benefited those who are more affluent in society. Health inequalities and the differences between population groups have received considerable interest from governments. This chapter will discuss the nature of health inequalities and the various explanations for their existence.

Learning outcomes

By the end of this chapter you will be able to:

- describe major social, economic and environmental influences on health
- define health inequalities
- understand the challenges of addressing health inequalities
- describe the role of the nurse in tackling health inequalities.

Inequalities in health

A health inequality is a term that describes differences between population groups according to socio-economic status, geographical area, ethnicity, age or gender, health status and access to and use of health services.

There are three types of health inequalities:

(1) inequality of access to health care, e.g. refugees or homeless people often have difficulty in obtaining access to primary health care services, such as registering with a general practitioner (GP)
(2) inequalities in health outcomes, e.g. there is a six year difference in life expectancy at birth across boroughs in London
(3) inequalities in the determinants of health, e.g. education, employment and housing can all have an influence on health status.

The determinants of health are a range of personal, social, economic and environmental factors that determine the health status of individuals and populations. Dahlgren and Whitehead's model (1991) (see Chapter 2 page 14) identifies these factors and shows them as layers of influence. These layers of influence include individual lifestyles but also social support, working conditions, education, housing and the physical environment. A wealth of research has shown the relationship between socio-economic status and health status in most Western countries, e.g. (MacIntyre, 1997). People from lower socio-economic groups have much poorer health than those in other groups. This is evident in relation to disease prevalence, life expectancy and infant mortality.

Figure 3.1 illustrates the relationship between occupational class and life expectancy and clearly demonstrates that the higher occupational groups have greater longevity than the lower occupational groups. Significantly, women fare best overall with women from professional groups living into their mid 80s, whereas women from the lowest occupational group living up to their mid 70s.

Table 3.1 illustrates how belonging to a lower socio-economic group may influence the health status of the individual. Major causes of death and illness in the UK – cancer, coronary heart disease (CHD), stroke, diabetes, accidents and deaths by suicide are closely linked to socio-economic status and people's access and availability to health service provision.

Table 3.2 illustrates the relationship between health status and wider factors in the individual's living conditions such as their housing, employment and living conditions.

Nurses should be aware of the inequalities experienced by certain population groups due to the care they receive. Black and minority ethnic groups for example, may also have difficulties in access to

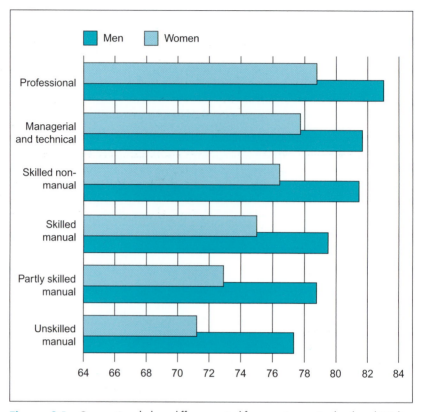

Figure 3.1 Occupational class differences in life expectancy, England and Wales, 1997–1999. Reproduced with permission from Social determinants of health: the solid facts (2nd ed.). Copenhagen, WHO Regional Office for Europe, 2003.

primary care, referral to hospital or community health services (Nazroo, 2001):

- out-patient attendance rates are lower for some Black and ethnic minority groups
- African-Caribbean men have high in-patient admission rates for schizophrenia
- South Asians have lower rates of GP consultation for mental health problems (http://www.lho.org.uk).

One major access barrier to health care for first generation migrants is language difference. For some groups, cultural differences in the perception of ill-health and lack of knowledge about the availability and range of health services can inhibit or delay their access to care until conditions become more serious. There is some evidence of this in rela-

Table 3.1 Health inequalities.

CHD	The death rate from CHD is three times higher among unskilled manual men of working age than among professional men
Obesity	28% of women in social class V (unskilled) are obese, compared to 14% in social class I (professional)
Accidents	Manual workers make up 42% of the workforce but account for 72% of reportable work-related injuries
	Children in social class V are five times more likely to suffer accidental death than children in social class I
Residential fire deaths	Residential fire deaths are 15 times more common for children in social class V compared to children in social class I
Mental health	Unskilled working men are almost four times more likely to commit suicide than their professional counterparts. Suicide rates in semi-skilled and manual unskilled workers are twice as high as the professional group

Source: DoH (2002)

Table 3.2 The impact of social factors on health.

Population indicators	Relevance to health
Unemployment	Associated with morbidity, injuries, poisoning and premature death, particularly CHD. Also associated with depression, anxiety, self-harm and suicide
Educational attainment: percentage of pupils achieving five general Certificate of Secondary Education (GCSE) grades A–C	Education reduces risk of unemployment and poverty which have a negative effect on health
Proportion of homes judged to be unfit to live in	Can cause or contribute to ill-health or injury and exacerbate existing conditions, e.g. through damp, cold, poor design or bad lighting
Burglary rate per 1000 population	The factors that affect the local crime rate also seem to affect health. Crime can also affect health indirectly through feeling unsafe

Source: Greater London Authority (2005)

tion to CHD in South Asian groups. 'Cultural competence' is the term used to describe services perceived by Black and minority ethnic users as being in harmony with their cultural and religious beliefs. As a result cultural competence training is becoming widespread (Chandra, 1996).

Activity

Why is it important for a nurse to know the socio-economic status
   of their patient?
What information needs to be collected to determine the social
   conditions in which your patients live?

Nurses need to be aware of the type of housing and the environment
their patients live in, their means of social support, their income,
employment status and their access to healthy affordable food and
leisure activities. This information will enable the nurse to plan care
to meet the needs of their patients and address gaps in service provision. Information about a patient's social situation will enable the nurse
not only to address their individual health needs but also address the
health needs of the wider community.

Explaining health inequalities

There have been many attempts to explain why ill-health is socially
patterned and there is no one answer. It is often claimed that
people on low incomes are more likely to lead unhealthy lifestyles
which results in poorer health status but there are many other
explanations:

Life course explanation

This explanation for health inequalities suggests that there are cumulative effects over the life course of an individual of material and psychosocial hazards and that these effects explain observed differences
in health and life expectancy. According to Kawachi *et al* (2000) life
course explanations are believed to have three pathways that are
relevant to health status:

(1)   The underlying effect of the early life environment affects the
      health of the adult, irrespective of other health behaviour or influ-
      ences on health. If for example, the mother smoked during her
      pregnancy, or was exposed to passive smoking during her preg-
      nancy this may have a detrimental effect on the health of the fetus
      in utero. Low birth-weight has been shown to be associated with
      health outcomes 50 years later in respect of CHD, stroke and
      respiratory disease mortality.
(2)   The early life environment of the individual will shape the indi-
      vidual's life course and in turn will affect their health status over
      time. A less advantaged family background is linked to worse
      education results, worse housing, job insecurity or unemployment
      and low work autonomy. Pre-school education programmes have

been shown to be related to later health through educational achievement, adult income and home ownership.

(3) The cumulative effects of being exposed to a health damaging environment, as well as the intensity and duration of that exposure can adversely affect the health status of the individual. For example, if the adult had been exposed over the course of their life time to a hazardous or unhealthy environment it could increase their likelihood of dying from cancer, CHD, strokes or respiratory illness.

Some conditions such as strokes, asthma and cancer of the stomach may be determined by early childhood circumstances, whereas, conditions such as deaths from lung cancer, accidents and violent attacks are more likely to be determined by the life course of the adult. The 1958 birth cohort study provides information on a sample of individuals as they grow older. Analysis of the data reveals childhood factors such as low birth-weight and height are linked to socio-economic circumstances. Childhood is also important in determining the later health status of the individual, as this is a period of dynamic global development, i.e. physical, social, intellectual and psychological. Therefore the individual will be more sensitive to environmental influences on health (Graham and Power, 2004).

Activity

Think of a patient that you have provided care for who has a long-term health condition, e.g. diabetes, hypertension or a stroke.

Reflecting on their medical history, what life events or circumstances do you think may have contributed to their current health status?

What actions could have been taken during their childhood to prevent their poor health status in adulthood?

Materialist/structural explanation

The materialist/structural explanation for health inequalities suggests that the health of the individual is determined by socio-economic and structural factors which contribute to the levels of poverty and deprivation experienced by the individual. Put simply it is the situation in which the individual lives which will determine their health. Those who are materially deprived are more likely to be exposed to poor housing conditions, environmental and work hazards, accidents at home, work and on the road and find it difficult to sustain a healthy life (Lynch *et al*, 2000).

In order to understand the relationship between socio-economic status and health we need to understand definitions of poverty, the scale of poverty and how poverty affects health. Poverty can be defined as absolute poverty or relative poverty. Absolute poverty for example would be the inability to meet your basic human needs such as access to food, shelter, warmth and safety (Kawachi *et al*, 2000). Relative poverty is determined by the standards of the rest of the society in which the individual lives. Although a person's basic needs may be met, they may be unable to afford any social participation. This inability to participate in the activities that enhance health such as community activities or social events is called social exclusion and has been used to describe those excluded from typically normal society. If people are socially excluded for any length of time they are more likely to suffer from a range of physical health problems, e.g. such as CHD, as well as social and emotional health stress and depression, marital breakdown and addiction to drugs and alcohol (WHO, 2003).

The individual's ability to socially engage with others and to make healthy choices will be determined by many factors including their disposable income. A study by Morris *et al* (2000) established that the minimum wage would not facilitate the ability to make healthy choices or socially engage with others.

Case study 3.1: Minimum income for healthy living

A study by Morris *et al* (2000) aimed to identify the minimal costs that a single, healthy, working man aged 18–30 years needed for running a home, disposable income and other basic necessities required for healthy living. This included food, clothing, accommodation, heating and social activities.

The information was obtained from ad hoc surveys and figures from the national Family Expenditure Survey. The study found that in 1999 the minimum costs needed to meet the above criteria were £131.86 per week. The national minimum wage in 1999 was £3.00 per hour/£105.84 per week for men aged 18–21 years; or £3.60 per hour/£121.12 per week for men aged 22 years. These figures were based on men working a 38 hour week.

In order for a person to earn enough money to live a healthy life (i.e. £131.86) an 18–21 year old man would have to work 51 hours per week and men aged 22 years and over would have to work 42.5 hours per week.

Behavioural/cultural explanation

This explanation for health inequalities will be very familiar to most health and social care professionals and has been that most favoured by successive governments. In this explanation for health inequalities it is suggested that the health of the individual is determined by behaviour such as:

- smoking
- drinking excessive amounts of alcohol
- being physically inactive
- consuming high levels of refined foods
- not using preventative health care services such as antenatal clinics, family planning clinics, immunisation/vaccination clinics or screening programmes.

All of these behaviours are linked to subsequent morbidity and mortality and are more common amongst lower social classes. Smoking among adults in the UK continues to be much more prevalent amongst manual groups compared with middle class people who are more likely to be able to quit. Risky health behaviours such as drug taking or drinking excessively are also much more common amongst lower social groups. A simple explanation might suggest irresponsibility or a lack of information on health risks on the part of the individual. However, research has shown that such behaviours are a response to social situations such as unemployment, social upheaval and stress. People use addictive behaviours such as cigarette smoking, drug taking and drinking excessive amounts of alcohol to 'numb the pain of harsh economic and social conditions' (WHO, 2003).

Scenario

Sandra is a single unsupported parent, living in a third floor council flat, with three children under five years and with very little disposable income. Sandra visits her GP several times in the course of three months complaining that her children have recurrent chest infections and her middle child has glue ear.

It is noted by her GP that Sandra is a heavy smoker and consequently her children are passive smokers. The GP tells Sandra that unless she stops smoking and attends the smoking cessation clinic run by the practice nurse she will not give her any more repeat prescriptions for antibiotics for chest infections for her children. When challenged about her smoking and faced with unfilled prescriptions Sandra becomes defensive and leaves the surgery angry and upset.

Is the ill-health of Sandra's children her fault?

How could the GP and practice nurse support Sandra in light of her current health behaviour?

What are the other influences on health that the GP and practice nurse need to be aware of?

What might be the problem of adopting a behavioural explanation of health inequalities to account for your patient's poor health?

This health behaviour on the part of Sandra may seem irresponsible and reckless, but faced with a life full of difficult decisions and a lack of choices and resources, it may be that smoking is health enhancing to Sandra's mental health, be it at the expense of the physical health of both her and her children (Graham, 1993).

It is too simplistic to assume that smoking is entirely a result of Sandra's irresponsible or reckless behaviour. Sandra's health behaviour could be as a result of her understanding of health, education or expectations. This blaming the victim approach can be very unhelpful for the nurse and patient as it may influence the way nurses respond to or care for patients – and it may mean patients defer seeking care and attention because they are afraid of being judged.

Psychosocial explanations

Stress can contribute to ill-health. The Whitehall II Study (Marmot *et al*, 1991) examined the reasons for the social gradient in health and disease, i.e. that higher occupational groups were less likely to suffer from CHD than lower occupational groups. This study highlighted the fact that health inequalities can occur because of the way work is organised and the work climate, i.e. those with a lack of autonomy, a lot of monotony and fewer relationships with superiors are more likely to experience stress at work. The more valued and in control people feel, the less likely they are to suffer from CHD, diabetes and metabolic syndrome.

Wilkinson (1997) argues that the psychosocial effects of social position account for the major part of health inequalities. It is the relationship between income, social position and health that is associated with an increased risk of CHD, stroke, hypertension, obesity and duodenal ulcers. Therefore if an individual is relatively poor in comparison to others within their society they are more likely to be at risk of developing any of these conditions. This may be a result of chronic stress and the physiological response to this stress, e.g. increased secretion of cortisol, elevated blood pressure, a change in the ratio of high-density and low-density lipoproteins, and a suppressed immune system. The psychological effects of stress which could lead to increased risk of developing the diseases and conditions can be buffered by social capital and networks, such as greater equality and group membership (WHO, 2003).

In order to enhance the psychological health of patients and address the effects of stress because of their feelings of helplessness, nurses need to encourage a sense of belonging, control and inclusion.

In order to make patients feel valued and included, it is important for the nurse to devise individual care plans that take into account patients' cultural, social and psychological needs as well as their physical health needs. By planning care jointly with patients i.e. that takes

> **Activity**
>
> How can the nurse ensure that their patients feel valued and included when they are admitted to the ward?
> How can this help the nurse to address health inequalities?

on board their expressed needs, values and beliefs, the nurse will be demonstrating a commitment to tackling health inequalities.

So far we have considered possible explanations for health inequalities and concluded that health inequalities could be due to:

- Life course explanations which suggest that the health status of the individual is determined by the environment that the individual is exposed to in utero to adulthood. Therefore those experiencing adverse economic conditions in early life are likely to be even more disadvantaged in adulthood.
- Materialist explanations of health inequalities suggest that the socio-economic background of the individual, the distribution of wealth and the impact of poverty influences the health status and wellbeing of the individual, thus accounting for the poorer health of lower socio-economic groups.
- Behavioural explanations of health inequalities suggest that it is the health behaviour of the individual such as smoking, physical inactivity, drinking in excess or eating an unhealthy diet, which will determine the health status of the individual and that these behaviours are more common in lower socio-economic groups.
- Psychosocial explanations which suggest that stress at home or work can contribute to long term ill-health.

Tackling health inequalities

There is much reference in current policy and legislation to tackling the root causes of ill-health and reference is made to 'upstream' measures. As we saw in Chapter 2 this refers to a move away from simply 'patching-up' people presenting for health care ('down stream'), to thinking about what or who is responsible for their health in the first place (upstream).

Although tackling health inequalities is now a major part of health roles and public policy, Conservative Governments of the 1980s and 90s refused to acknowledge the issue of health inequalities and much later, in the mid 1990s used the term 'variations in health' as a means of explaining health inequalities. Concern about the differences in health experienced by different population groups arose again on the election of the New Labour Government in 1997 who commissioned an independent inquiry into health inequalities known as the Acheson Report (1998). This report not only reiterated the findings of the Black Report (1980) and the later Health Divide (1987) (Townsend and Davidson, 1987) but also more worryingly highlighted the growing divide between the health of the poorest and wealthiest in society. Acheson (1998) was commissioned to review the evidence on health inequalities in England and provide an in depth analysis of a range of inequality including age, gender and ethnicity in addition to poverty.

The Acheson Report (1998) found that overall the nation's health had improved and morbidity and mortality rates from infectious diseases had made impressive improvements, with the health of the most advantaged groups making the most dramatic improvement. However, health inequalities had actually increased between rich and poor since the Black Report was published in 1980.

Acheson (1998) argued that health inequalities can be explained by socio-economic causes such as income, education, employment, environment and lifestyle and that these influences on health should be addressed by Government in terms of policy development. This would entail tackling poverty by establishing a national minimum wage and changes in taxation and state benefits allowances, better education, more employment opportunities, improved housing and the living environment, tackling pollution and improving nutrition. Acheson (1998) specifically focused on the needs of mothers, children and families, young people and adults of working age and older adults. Acheson (1998) also acknowledged the needs of Black and minority ethnic groups.

Acheson (1998) outlined three areas as priorities in tackling health inequalities:

- policies that were likely to impact on health should be evaluated with regard to their impact on health inequalities
- priority should be given to the health of families with children
- there should be further steps taken to address income inequalities and improve the living conditions of the deprived households.

In response to the Acheson Report (1998) and other evidence the Government introduced many policies aimed at tackling health inequalities including:

Area-based health programmes

These are part of the Government's *Improvement, Expansion & Reform: The Next Three Years (2003–2006)* (DoH, 2003). These programmes aim to reduce health inequalities across different groups and across different areas in the country, but initially aims to focus on reducing the gap in infant mortality and life expectancy at birth and reducing rates of teenage pregnancy.

Local strategic partnerships

These aim to form strategic partnerships between the statutory agencies and the local community to tackle health inequalities at a local level by looking for local solutions to address inequalities.

Neighbourhood renewal

This aims to tackle health inequalities by targeting the most disadvantaged areas and introducing a range of activities to reduce crime and deprivation such as improving housing, improving leisure and recreation facilities, job creation schemes, local community action projects and neighbourhood watch schemes (see www.neighbourhood.gov.uk).

Improving health status across the life course

Includes policies and programmes aimed at improving the early development of the fetus and child to increase their likelihood of a healthy adulthood, e.g.

Promoting cessation of smoking in pregnancy

In the UK approximately 35% of women smoke prior to pregnancy and about 5–10% will stop during pregnancy. The effects of smoking in pregnancy include a pre-term labour, a low birth-weight baby, fetal inter-uterine growth retardation and maternal high blood pressure. Interventions include behavioural support through cessation groups and telephone counselling and biochemical support through Nicotine Replacement Therapy.

Promoting breast feeding

The Infant Feeding Survey (DoH, 2000a) found that although 74% of first time mothers initially breast feed their babies, there is a steep social class gradient ranging from 51% in women from social class V to 91% in women from social class I. The survey also found that breast feeding was age related ranging from 46% for teenage mothers to 78% for women aged over 30 years. The Breast Feeding Initiative aims to support women to breast feed by giving one-to-one support, small group discussions and promoting a breast feeding friendly environment in shops and restaurants (DoH, 2000a).

Healthy Start scheme

This was introduced during 2005 to address the nutritional needs of pregnant women and children by providing vouchers for those on a low income which could be exchanged for milk, fresh fruit or vegetables (see www.healthystart.nhs.uk).

Childhood nutrition programmes

Research shows that most children in the UK eat too much saturated fat, sugar and salt. Children on average eat only two portions of fruit and vegetables a day and children from social class V tend to eat 50% less fruit and vegetables than those from social class I. The consumption of carbonated drinks in children aged 4–18 years was equivalent to five cans a day for boys and four cans a day for girls (DoH, 2000b). The national school fruit and vegetable scheme. This gives all children aged four to six years, in local education authority schools, one piece of free fruit or vegetable each school day (www.5aday.nhs.uk).

These initiatives aim to tackle health inequalities across the life course and target specific high risk groups. Of course such policies and programmes may not be enough to enable people faced with difficult circumstances and limited resources to make the healthier choice.

Global perspective on tackling health inequalities

So far we have focussed on public health and health promotion policies and initiatives in the UK which were developed to tackle health inequalities. However, it is important to note that these policies and initiatives were developed as part of a global perspective aimed at tackling the health inequalities of disadvantaged groups across the world. The lead organisation charged with developing health care policy is the World Health Organization (WHO). As part of their public health policy development role in 2004 the WHO commissioned global research to investigate the issues behind health inequalities.

The WHO (2004) found that there is evidence of health inequalities from across nations in relation to infant mortality rates and across the life span. For example, the infant mortality rate for American-Indians and Alaskan natives is almost double that of White Americans. Mortality rates from cancer are 30% higher for African-Americans than for White Americans (Smedley *et al*, 2003). In Northern Ireland women from social class V were more than 60% more likely to experience some form of neurotic disorder than women from higher social classes. (Ministry for Health Social Services and Public Safety, 2002).

Activity

Why is it important for nurses to have a global perspective on health?

How will this global perspective influence your everyday practice?

The world is becoming smaller and the effects of globalisation are felt worldwide, for example:

- the impact of enterprises such as food chains and restaurants on the diet and health of communities (Beaglehole and Yach, 2003)
- the effects of the tobacco industry specifically targeting previously untapped markets and younger smokers (American Health Association, 2006)
- the arms trade and sports industries are increasingly using workforces composed of children to manufacture their goods (American Public Health Association, 2001).

Nurses have an important and influential role as public health advocates to speak out against health damaging and irresponsible behaviour on the part of industry. Brundtland (1999) cited by the RCN (1999) argues in relation to tobacco control that:

> *Nurses have many opportunities to play a leadership role in combating the tobacco epidemic. Nurses throughout the world have access to the population at all levels of the health care system, and enjoy a high degree of public trust. Indeed, there are several examples of nurses successfully initiating and implementing tobacco prevention and treatment programmes with specific target populations, such as school children, pregnant women and people recovering from cardiac diseases and cancer. The International Council of Nurses has urged nurses to get involved at all levels of tobacco control: prevention, cessation, and policy, encouraging them to be at the forefront of tobacco control at the local, national and international level, building partnerships with other professional and advocacy groups, governmental and non-governmental organizations.*

The role of the nurse in tackling health inequalities

Improving access and availability to health care involves the nurse firstly acknowledging that disadvantaged groups may not have the same access to good quality health care provision as more affluent groups. The nurse should aim to ensure equal access by: developing explicit guideline referrals; employing positive discrimination principles such as prioritising disadvantaged groups; making sure services are more accessible through such measures as out of hours clinics; screening high risk groups and; ensuring that health information is accessible for high risk and disadvantaged groups. Evidence suggests that these approaches and interventions targeting disadvantaged groups are proven to be effective at addressing health inequalities (Patterson and Judge, 2002). The nurse also needs to acknowledge that patients do not have equal opportunities to address their health problems.

Nurses should involve their patients as much as possible in planning their care to ensure that the care plan meets the patient's needs. Other considerations for the nurses include ensuring that in their everyday dealing with their patients that they adopt anti-discriminatory practice principles which include, being flexible, including the views of marginalised and excluded groups, challenging existing stereotypes and practices and reflecting on organisational structures and the way that structure may reinforce health inequalities (Burke and Harrison, 1998).

The nurse may also try to influence policy both nationally or locally to tackle health inequalities. This may include writing to policy makers to highlight issues which promote health inequalities. Evidence suggests that lobbying as a tool for change can be effective – some researchers for example believe that lobbying from the public health field brought about an acknowledgement by the Conservative Government regarding variations in health, as the Government had previously refused to acknowledge that health inequalities existed (Baggott, 2000). There is currently an active campaign to keep the National Health Service (NHS) public (www.keepournhspublic. com) and nurses and international organisations such as UNICEF have successfully lobbied international formula milk companies in relation to the companies' promotion of bottle feeding in developing countries.

Partnership working involves the nurse working collaboratively with other agencies to form local strategies to tackle health inequalities. Nurses may join forces with social workers, community workers, charities and leisure services to devise projects that tackle health inequalities. Evidence suggests that the multidisciplinary approach is an important factor in the success of interventions that improve the health of disadvantaged groups (Arblaster et al, 1996). For example, community nurses have successfully collaborated with organisations such as the Child Accident Prevention Trust to produce a training programme and resources for health visitors and other community nurses to use to tackle children's accidents at home.

Promoting health enhancing behaviours involves the nurse participating in health promotion programmes such as smoking cessation groups. These programmes would be targeted at disadvantaged groups and would aim to tackle health damaging behaviour. Evidence shows that these programmes have some success in tackling health inequalities, e.g. reducing smoking rates in disadvantaged groups or increasing breast feeding initiation and maintenance (Lowey et al, 2002; NHS, 2000). One criticism of this approach is the top down focus, i.e. addressing the individual's behaviour and failing to look bottom up, i.e. the causes of health inequalities such as policies, poor housing, unemployment, social class, age and ethnicity (Evans, 2003).

Summary

This chapter has considered some of the evidence that demonstrates that ill-health is concentrated in the poorer sections of society. It has outlined some policy initiatives which aim to improve the health of those living in disadvantaged communities. Community nurses are ideally placed to promote health in these communities as they have good access to families. But all nurses need to be aware of the impact of social factors on the health of their patients.

Further reading and resources

Acheson D. (1998) *Independent Inquiry into Inequalities and Health* London, The Stationery Office.

A summary of recent evidence of health inequalities that is readable and policy oriented.

World Health Organization. (2003) *Social Determinants of Health. The Solid Facts* 2nd ed. WHO Copenhagen, (www.who.dk/document).

A clear and accessible explanation for health inequalities worldwide.

London is one of nine regional Public Health Observatories set up in England in 2001 by the Department of Health. London Health Observatory takes the national lead role in monitoring health inequalities, ethnicity and tobacco.

Health Start: www.healthystart.nhs.uk
London Health Observatory: http://www.lho.org.uk
NHS–5 a day: www.5aday.nhs.uk
NHS–keep our NHS public: www.keepournhspublic.com

References

Acheson D. (1998) *Independent Inquiry into Inequalities and Health*. London, The Stationery Office.

American Health Association (2006) *Tobacco Industry's Targeting of Youth, Minorities and Women*. AHA, Washington.

American Public Health Association (2001) *Global Trade and Global Health: APHA Perspectives*. APHA, Washington.

Arblaster L. Lambert M. and Entwistle V. (1996) A Systematic Review of the Effectiveness of Health Service Interventions Aimed at Reducing Inequalities in Health, *Journal of Health Services Research and Policy*, **1**, 2, 93–103.

Baggott R. (2000) *Public Health: Policy and Politics*. Basingstoke, Palgrave Macmillan.

Beaglehole R. and Yach D. (2003) Globalisation and The Prevention and Control Of Non-Communicable Disease: The Neglected Chronic Diseases of Adults, *The Lancet*, **362**, 903–8.

Brundtland G. (1999) cited by the RCN (1999) *Clearing the Air* RCN, London.

Burke B. and Harrison P. (1998) Anti-Oppressive Practice. In Adams R. Dominelli L. and Payne M. (Eds.) *Social Work: Themes, Issues and Critical Debates*. Basingstoke, Palgrave Macmillan.

Chandra J. (1996) *Facing up to difference* Kings Fund, London.

Dahlgren G. and Whitehead M. (1991) *Policies and Strategies to Promote Social Equity in Health*. Stockholm, Institute for Futures Studies.

Department of Health (2000a) *Infant Feeding Survey*. The Stationery Office, London.

Department of Health (2000b) *National Diet & Nutrition Survey*. The Stationery Office, London.

Department of Health (2002) *Tackling Health Inequalities 2002 Cross Cutting Review*. The Stationery Office, London.

Department of Health (2003) *Improvement, Expansion & Reform: The Next Three Years (2003–2006)*. The Stationery Office, London.

Evans D. (2003) New Directions in Tackling Inequalities. In Orme J. Powell J. Taylor P. Harrison T. and Grey M. (Eds.) *Public Health for the 21st Century New Perspectives on Policy, Participation and Practice*. Maidenhead, Open University.

Graham H. (1993) *When Life's a Drag: Women, Smoking and Disadvantage*. HMSO, London.

Greater London Authority (2005) *Health in London: Review of the London Health Strategy High Level Indicators*. Health Commission, London.

Graham H. and Power C. (2004) *Childhood Disadvantage and Adult Health: A Lifecourse Framework*. London, Health Development Agency.

Kawachi I. Subramanian SV. and Almeida-Filho N. (2000) A Glossary for Health Inequalities, *Journal of Epidemiology and Community Health*, **54**, 885–9.

Lowey H. Fullard B. Tocque K. and Bellis M. (2002) *Are Smoking Cessation Services Reducing Health Inequalities in Health?* Liverpool, North West Public Health Observatory.

Lynch J. Davey Smith G. Kaplan G. House J. (2000) Income Inequality and Mortality: Importance to Health of Individual Income, Psychological Environment or Material Conditions, *British Medical Journal*, **44**, 6, 723–45.

MacIntyre S. (1997) The Black Report and Beyond: What are the issues? *Social Science and Medicine*, **44**, 723–45.

Marmot MG. Davey Smith G. Stansfield SA. Patel C. North F. Head J. (1991) Health Inequalities among British Civil Servants: The Whitehall II Study, *Lancet*, **331**, 1387–93.

Ministry for Health Social Services and Public Safety (2002) cited by the WHO (2004) *Closing the Health Inequalities Gap: An International Perspective*, WHO, Venice.

Morris JN. Donkin AJM. Wonderling DP. Wilkinson P. and Dowler EA. (2000) A Minimum Income for Healthy Living, *Journal Epidemiology and Community Health*, **54**, 885–9.

National Health Service (2000) Promoting the Initiation of Breastfeeding, *Effective Healthcare Bulletin*, **6**, 2, NHS Centre for Reviews and Dissemination, York.

Nazroo J. (2001) *Ethnicity Class & Health*. London, Policy Studies Institute.

Patterson I. and Judge K. (2002) Equality of Access to Healthcare. In Mackenbach J. and Baker M. (Eds.) *Reducing Inequalities in Health: A European Perspective*. London, Routledge.

Smedley BD. Smith AY. and Nelson AR. (2003) *Unequal Treatment: Confronting Racial and Ethnic Disparities in Health Care*. New York, National Academic Press.

Townsend P. and Davidson N. (1987) *Inequalities in Health: The Health Divide*. London, Penguin Books.

World Health Organization. (2003) *Social Determinant of Health. The Solid Facts* 2nd ed. WHO, Copenhagen.

World Health Organisation (2004) *Closing the Health Inequalities Gap: An International Perspective*. WHO, Venice.

Wilkinson R. (1997) *Unhealthy Societies: the Afflictions of Inequality*. London, Routledge.

Approaches to Promoting Health

Susie Sykes

Introduction

This chapter will consider in more detail the different perspectives that practitioners have towards health and the ways in which these may influence how nurses interpret the conditions that patients present with. There are a number of different approaches to health promotion that may be adopted according to the perspective of health that is held, the objectives that need to be met or political persuasion. This chapter will look at medical approaches to health promotion which focus on: preventing disease and treating illness; behavioural approaches which concentrate on strategies for changing people's behaviour in favour of healthier lifestyles and; socio-environmental approaches which aim to effect change on the wider social and cultural environment within which health is constructed. Students will be encouraged to consider how different theoretical approaches to health promotion can be applied through their roles as nurses.

Learning outcomes

By the end of this chapter you will be able to:

- describe the difference between biomedical, behavioural and social approaches to health promotion
- describe different aspects of health promotion in relation to theoretical models available
- use an understanding of different health promotion models and theories in order to design and plan health promotion interventions that can be used in the role of a nurse.

Perspectives of health

There are a number of ways of conceptualising and understanding health. These different perspectives consider health and prioritise determinants of health in various ways. They therefore go on to foster different approaches to responding to health issues. This chapter will focus on three of these perspectives:

- biomedical
- behavioural
- socio-environmental.

As we saw in Chapter 2, health is often viewed as the absence of disease and disability which is achieved largely through clinical measures. For those operating within this framework, health is seen as being determined primarily by physiological risk factors. A behavioural perspective, on the other hand, acknowledges the importance of this medical model of health but sees health as being influenced by the way in which people live their lives. This perspective sees lifestyle as key in determining health alongside physiological risks. Others however, take biomedical and behavioural perspectives further and include within their definition of health social quality of life. This socio-environmental perspective sees health as being primarily influenced by the social and economic environment within which people live and the constraints and opportunities such structural factors create. People's economic situation, housing conditions, education and employment for example, all impact on people's health and contribute to how easily they are able to take on board health messages and adopt healthier lifestyles. Many of these structural issues may be beyond a patient's immediate control.

Consider, for example, a patient who is suffering from Coronary Heart Disease (CHD). The condition can be interpreted differently according to the three perspectives of health that have been outlined above. According to Naidoo and Wills (2000):

- a biomedical perspective would focus on CHD as being the result of physiological factors, hypertension, a build up of arterial plaque or genetic influences
- a behavioural perspective would focus on CHD as being the result of lifestyle factors such as smoking, high fat diet, lack of exercise or high levels of alcohol consumption
- a socio-environmental perspective would consider issues such as stress caused by situational factors, e.g. employment, poverty, isolation and family conflict.

Most professionals do not operate solely within the confines of just one of these perspectives but are likely to be influenced by one perspective more than the others. It is important to reflect upon and understand one's own perspective in order to consider why we respond to issues and prioritise actions in the way that we do.

Activity

- Reflect on which of the three perspectives of health (biomedical, behavioural or socio-environmental) influences your thinking most when you are considering a patient's condition.
- Why does this perspective influence your thinking more than others?
- Are there times when more than one perspective influences your thinking?
- What difference would viewing a patient's condition from a different health perspective make?

For those working in a hospital environment with emphasis on clinical targets and outcomes, the biomedical perspective of health can often dominate a nurse's thinking. Taking time to reflect upon how behavioural and socio-environmental factors may also have played a part in a patient's condition, enables the nurse to identify appropriate and sustainable health promotion responses.

Approaches to health promotion

The particular perspective of health that is held directly influences the approaches that are taken in health promotion interventions and will affect the way strategies are planned and implemented.

Biomedical approaches to health promotion

A biomedical approach to health promotion has as its primary focus the prevention of ill-health and disease rather than prioritising the promotion of positive health and wellbeing. In working to achieve this, a biomedical approach focuses fundamentally on addressing physiological risk factors. It is concerned essentially with clinical interventions to prevent disease and tends to be expert-led, i.e. initiated and led by professionals rather than by the patient. Typical interventions are those that target whole populations or which are focused on high risk target groups and would include activities such as immunisation and screening programmes. As such, interventions tend to be based on and driven by epidemiological evidence and are usually target driven. For example, the annual influenza immunisation campaigns are based on epidemiological data and target certain groups such as those over 65 years, and those in particular clinical risk groups. The campaign has epidemiologically driven targets including the immunisation of over 70% of people over 65 years (DoH, 2005).

Interventions that fit within this approach often receive higher recognition and credibility than other approaches as they fit within a scientific framework that is dominant within a Western medical model of health. They are usually assessed in terms of levels of morbidity and mortality and other clinical indicators. The clinical nature of this approach to health promotion means that it fits comfortably within a hospital setting and as a result can dominate how clinicians plan and implement health promotion initiatives.

Critics argue that an emphasis on this approach results in an over medicalisation of issues without considering the context of how people live their lives or taking into account the wider social, cultural and economic factors that contribute to and determine health.

Case study 4.1: National Health Service Breast Screening Programme (NHSBSP)

The NHSBSP was set up in 1998 to provide free breast screening every three years for all women in the UK aged 50 years or over. The aim of the programme is to reduce the death toll amongst women from breast cancer through early detection and treatment. Women are routinely invited for screening through their general practitioner (GP) and the programme screens an average of 1.5 million women every year. Research undertaken by the Department of Health (2006) concluded that 1400 lives are saved annually through the early detection of breast cancer by this scheme. This initiative is focused on preventing disease and does not include within its objectives promoting a positive sense of health and wellbeing.

Behavioural approaches to health promotion

Behavioural approaches to health promotion are based on a recognition of the impact that people's lifestyle and behaviour have on their health. Health promotion interventions based on this perspective seek to change people's behaviour and encourage the adoption of healthier lifestyles and therefore prevent ill-health. Their aims may however go further and include the promotion of positive health and wellbeing. This approach became more dominant through the 1970s and 80s as the impact of lifestyles on health became increasingly recognised (Lavarack, 2005).

The focus of behavioural approaches to health promotion may be educational – giving people accurate information about the impact of their behaviour on their health so that they are able to make informed choices about their lifestyle, e.g. nutritional information about what is required to ensure a healthy diet. It may however, go beyond the giving of information and include work to develop the skills and strategies that people require to implement and sustain changes in their lifestyle, e.g., cooking skills and strategies to develop menu options that appeal to all family members.

Behavioural-based interventions tend to be focused on individuals or small groups, although population-based health education campaigns that seek to change people's behaviour, such as media-based smoking or sexual health campaigns, also fit within this approach. The agenda and process of this approach tends to be expert-led although this is not always the case and negotiation with patients can occur. Hospital settings are often seen as appropriate settings within which to undertake a behavioural approach to health promotion, in part because of the high prestige and credibility of hospital staff giving an authority to behavioural and lifestyle messages (Johnson and Baum, 2001) and because patients can be targeted at a time when their health is at the forefront of their minds.

The effectiveness of this approach is however dependant on individuals being at a point at which they are ready and able to make changes in their behaviour. Critics claim that such interventions tend to focus on an individual's behaviour without looking more widely at the structural circumstances that influence those behaviours (Lavarack, 2004; Caraher, 1998). For example, interventions that encourage people to adopt a healthier diet and eat five portions of fruit and vegetables a day as recommended by the Department of Health's 5-A-Day programme (DoH, 2003), may not necessarily explore structural barriers to doing so. These may include: the cost of fresh food; public transport to out of town supermarkets where food might be cheaper and, media messages to children which promote fast food. Chapter 8 discusses the ways in which practitioners can promote healthy lifestyles without victim blaming and seeing the individual as solely responsible for their situation.

Scenario:
Initiating breastfeeding.

In an attempt to increase the numbers of new mothers breastfeeding their babies, a group of midwives might include a session in the antenatal classes on breastfeeding. The session may provide plenty of information on the benefits of breastfeeding for both the baby and the new mother and also demonstrate effective techniques. Leaflets might be made available that summarise the information given during the session. Women may also be provided with contact details of a breastfeeding specialist who they can contact after their baby is born if they feel they are experiencing difficulties breastfeeding and want additional support.

What limitations can you identify with this approach?

Such initiatives are based on the assumption that the main reasons why mothers do not breastfeed is a lack of information and under-standing of the benefits, such as increased resistance to infection, as well as a need for information on how to breastfeed successfully. It does not seek to address other barriers that mothers may face and which may be a more powerful reason why breastfeeding is not chosen. It does not, for example, look at cultural norms and negative attitudes towards breastfeeding that may make breastfeeding less acceptable and create barriers in some sections of the population. Research carried out in Scotland, for example, found that embarrassment, concern about other people's disapproval and fear of losing one's freedom and per-sonal identity all acted as barriers to women deciding to breastfeed (HEBS, 2001). It also does not look at difficulties faced by mothers who have to return to work soon after the birth of their baby.

Socio-environmental approaches to health promotion

Advocates of a socio-environmental approach to health promotion emphasise the view that medical and behavioural interventions should take place alongside interventions that address the wider structural social and economic factors that impact on the health of individuals, communities and populations. This approach is based on an argument that the determinants of health are highly complex and include indi-vidual, social, economic, cultural and environmental influences and as such require complex responses. The focus of this approach is about bringing change at a policy or structural level in order to create an environment in which it becomes both possible and realistic for indi-viduals to make and sustain healthy choices and lifestyles. Examples of this kind of approach are campaigns such as those carried out by *Which* ? (2005) and the Consumers Association (2002) for changes to food labelling regulations so that the nutritional value of food is more easily known to people, thus making it easier for people to choose healthier options.

Interventions that operate within this approach and which seek to address a number of the wider determinants of health may be complex, long term, require support at a strategic level and be dependant on intersectoral commitment. For this reason, many nurses may see it as being beyond their ability or remit to adopt this approach. It has been argued that nurses have, in the past, tended to adopt a limited, tradi-tional health education-based approach that focuses on the giving of information (Whitehead, 2005). While it is indeed difficult for a nurse to directly bring about large scale structural change through ward based hospital work, there are opportunities at every level to influence or lobby for structural change. This may include critical consciousness-raising among patients as part of a process of empowering patients to recognise social injustice and become active for change. Within this approach a nurse has the potential to become one part of a larger movement for change. It has been argued that in order to have a sustainable impact on the health of the communities within which they work, there is a need for nurses to be politically aware and develop broad policy analysis skills as an integral part of their professional development (Whitehead, 2003; Naidoo and Wills, 2005). In the previous chapter we discussed how nurses can tackle inequalities through nursing practice.

Case study 4.2: A specialist asthma nurse

A specialist asthma nurse describes how she can play a part in addressing the wider structural determinants of health:

In my capacity as a paediatric asthma nurse I was asked to go and review a three-year old boy in the children's ward who had been admitted with an asthma attack. I did all my usual education – what asthma is, looked at what things may have precipitated that attack, necessary treatments, inhaler techniques, management plan, etc. This also included looking at the home environment. During that time, the child's mother became very upset and told me about the damp and mould in their flat. The child's mother invited me to their home to see the damp for myself.

The flat was covered in damp and mould from an ongoing leak from the balcony above. She felt that she was getting nowhere with the council regarding being re-housed. This was wearing her down mentally and emotionally and she was finding it harder to cope with her son's illness. She reported feeling suicidal and unable to go on. I wrote a letter to the Housing Department stating the child's medical needs, enclosing a medical paper about the effects of damp housing, and also the psychological state of the mother and the possible impact that would be having on her ability to cope with her son's needs.

The family did get re-housed within quite a short space of time. The child's mother's mood changed after this and the child's asthma is much better controlled – I don't see him now. It is always difficult to determine direct cause and effect but we cannot look at any of these things in isolation and need to treat them as a whole within their family and environment.

Paediatric Asthma Nurse

While this intervention did not bring about policy change, it did impact on the implementation of a policy that influences the wider determinations of health. Ongoing involvement in this way has the potential to influence longer term policy review or development.

Table 4.1 Summary of perspectives of health and approaches to health promotion.

Perspective of health	Determinants of health viewed in terms of	Examples of health promotion interventions
Biomedical	• Physiological risk factors • Family history/genetic risk factors • Exposure to pathogens	• Clinical interventions • Immunisation and screening programmes • Drug treatments
Behavioural	Lifestyle and behaviour such as: • Smoking • Diet • Activity levels • Sexual activity • Stress levels	• Health education programmes • Campaigns • One-to-one advice • Small group work/self help groups
Socio-environmental	Social and economic environment e.g.: • Economic deprivation • Housing • Employment conditions • Low educational levels • Social exclusion and isolation	• Policy and legislation change • Advocacy • Lobbying and petitioning

Adapted from Ontario Health Promotion Resource System

There is overlap between these three different approaches and planned health promotion interventions may not sit solely within one of these perspectives. The type of intervention chosen will vary according to the circumstances and the objectives that need to be met. However, this provides a useful framework within which to consider the direction from which work is currently undertaken and the potential for it to be undertaken differently. Table 4.1 illustrates the three different perspectives on health.

Models of health promotion

The perspectives discussed represent broad approaches to health promotion but it is useful to go beyond this and look at more detailed models of health promoting activity. Models provide a theoretical framework through which to view health promotion as a whole and help us consider, not only how different perspectives of health can be actioned but also how our political philosophy, values and beliefs influence the way we develop and implement strategies for health promotion. They provide a tool for questioning practice and the assumptions that form the basis of practice. Through such models, a framework can be provided for developing new strategies (Katz et al, 2000). Theoretical models should, however, also be viewed critically. They are intended to support thinking but an over reliance on one particular model may close minds to alternative visions. It should also be remembered that they are not, unlike nursing models, a guide to what to do.

Activity

Consider health promotion interventions with the objectives of tackling obesity.

- What advantages and disadvantages exist in targeting health promotion interventions at:
  (a) Individuals, e.g. weight loss programmes or nutritional counselling?
  (b) Populations, e.g. local food cooperative schemes or campaigns to improve school meals?
- What advantages and disadvantages exist in health promotion interventions that are:
  (a) 'Top down', decided upon and led by professionals and experts (such as healthy eating campaigns)?
  (b) Negotiated with patients and based on principles of involvement and participation (such as weight loss programmes)?

Interventions targeted at individuals can be tailor-made and can be targeted at those most in need in a way that ensures they meet the specific needs of the individual. An individual focus assumes however that behaviour is voluntarily chosen or inherent in cultural or social norms. Population-based interventions mean that large numbers of people can be targeted but require rather general objectives that may not meet the specific needs of minority or vulnerable groups within that population.

Top down approaches to health promotion mean that work is based on usually epidemiological evidence of what most needs to be addressed and what has been found to work. This approach does not however allow patients the same degree of ownership and commitment that may come from a more negotiated and user-led approach.

Tannahill's model of health promotion

This model (Figure 4.1) was developed to illustrate the scope of health promotion (Downie et al, 1996). According to this model, health promo-

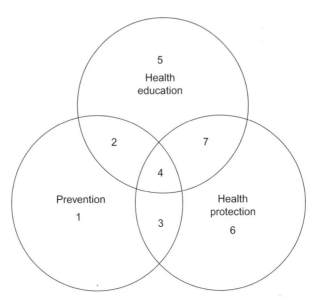

Figure 4.1   Tannahill model of health promotion. Reproduced with permission from Downie RS. Tannahill C. and Tannahill A. (1996) *Health Promotion, Models and Values* Oxford, Oxford University Press.

tion is made up of three overlapping areas; health education, health protection and prevention.

- Health education is defined as work to promote positive health and wellbeing and to prevent or reduce ill-health through the influencing of beliefs, attitudes and behaviours.
- Health protection includes regulatory work through legislative and policy-based interventions to protect the health and wellbeing of individuals, communities and populations.
- Prevention broadly refers to work through services to reduce the likelihood of poor health.

A feature of this model is that it distinguishes throughout between enhancing positive health and preventing ill-health and sees health promotion as aiming to undertake both these objectives.

Within the three overlapping circles there are seven different domains, each of which refers to a different type of activity and all of which form a part of what defines health promotion. Each of the domains is described in Table 4.2.

The Tannahill model is designed to present the different domains of health promotion without judgement of one being of greater value than another (Katz *et al*, 2000). It provides an explicit acknowledgement that there is overlap between the different activities that define health promotion. It does not represent within it different political

Table 4.2 Domains of health promotion activity within the Tannahill model.

Domain	Characteristics	Examples of typical interventions
(1) Prevention services	Programmes and services designed to prevent disease and ill-health	Immunisation screening programmes Nicotine replacement therapy
(2) Prevention health education	Education to influence lifestyles to prevent ill-health combined with encouragement to use prevention services	Smoking cessation advice in conjunction with the provision of nicotine replacement therapy
(3) Preventive health protection	Policies and regulation to prevent disease and ill-health	Fluoridation of water supplies to prevent dental health problems
(4) Health education of preventive health protection	Educating policy makers for the need for preventive regulations while educating a community to seek or accept changes	Lobbying for policies on seat belts
(5) Health education	Influencing behaviour on positive health grounds to encourage the development of healthy attributes including self-esteem and communication	Life skills and relationship training
(6) Positive health protection	Regulations and policies that promote positive health and wellbeing	Workplace smoking policy
(7) Health education for positive health protection	Educating policy makers for the need for positive health regulations while educating a community to accept or seek change.	Lobbying for a smoking ban in public places

philosophies that may underpin different approaches or explore the extent to which interventions may be participatory and negotiated or imposed and expert-led. The key to this model is also the fact that communication within the health promotion function is not limited to discussion with, or education of, patients. It also involves communication with and education of hospital management and policy makers

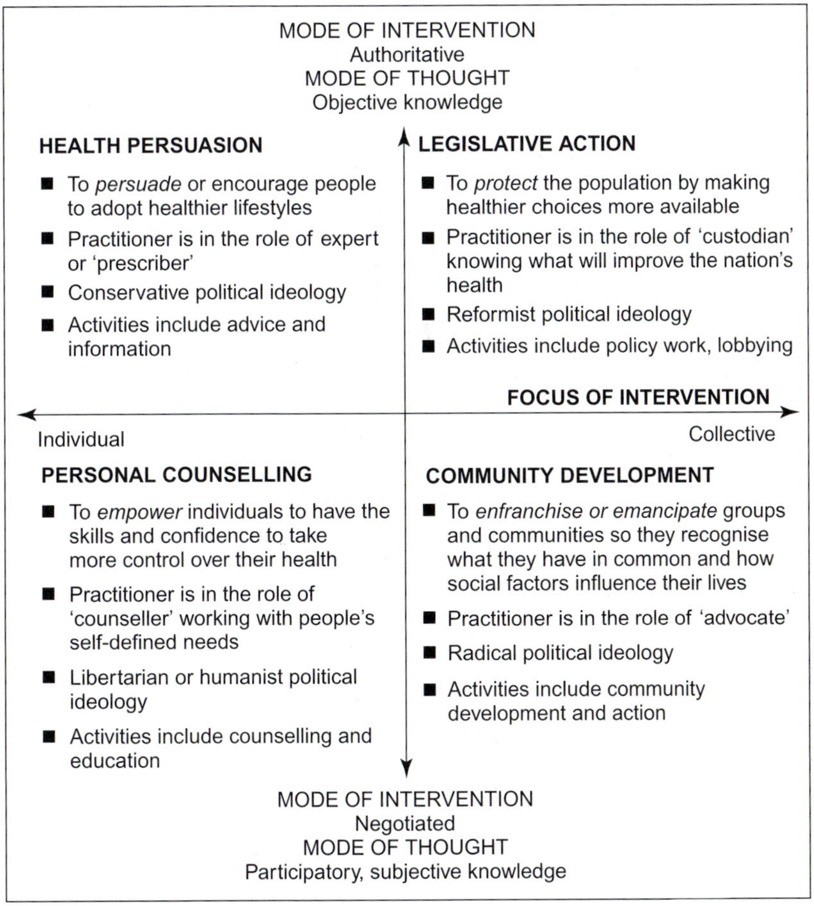

MODE OF INTERVENTION
Authoritative
MODE OF THOUGHT
Objective knowledge

HEALTH PERSUASION

- To *persuade* or encourage people to adopt healthier lifestyles
- Practitioner is in the role of expert or 'prescriber'
- Conservative political ideology
- Activities include advice and information

LEGISLATIVE ACTION

- To *protect* the population by making healthier choices more available
- Practitioner is in the role of 'custodian' knowing what will improve the nation's health
- Reformist political ideology
- Activities include policy work, lobbying

FOCUS OF INTERVENTION

Individual ← → Collective

PERSONAL COUNSELLING

- To *empower* individuals to have the skills and confidence to take more control over their health
- Practitioner is in the role of 'counseller' working with people's self-defined needs
- Libertarian or humanist political ideology
- Activities include counselling and education

COMMUNITY DEVELOPMENT

- To *enfranchise or emancipate* groups and communities so they recognise what they have in common and how social factors influence their lives
- Practitioner is in the role of 'advocate'
- Radical political ideology
- Activities include community development and action

MODE OF INTERVENTION
Negotiated
MODE OF THOUGHT
Participatory, subjective knowledge

Figure 4.2 Beattie's model of health promotion. Reprinted from Health Promotion: Foundations for Practice, Naidoo J. and Wills J. 2000, with permission from Elsevier.

(Latter, 2001). It is necessary for nurses to recognise this as part of their health promoting role if they are to move beyond the traditional confines of health education.

Beattie's model of health promotion

Beattie's model (Beattie, 1991) presents four quadrants of activity derived from two axes on a grid (Figure 4.2). The vertical axis represents modes of interventions that range from authoritarian, top down, expert-led interventions to bottom up, negotiated, participatory approaches to health promotion. It could be suggested that nurses have been traditionally associated with fairly authoritarian, top down interventions, but they also have the potential to play an important role in more participatory forms of health promotion (Scriven, 2005) as the following examples will demonstrate. The horizontal axis represents the focus of activities ranging from interventions targeting individuals, to those focused on tackling the social determinants of health. Again, the nurse's role is often seen to fit more comfortably with a focus on individuals despite a shifting emphasis to collective approaches within the field of health promotion (Whitehead, 2005). Within Beattie's model there are four spheres of health promotion activity:

- health persuasion
- legislative action
- personal counselling
- community development.

Health persuasion

Health persuasion activities involve an expert-led, top down approach that represents a rather paternalistic and conservative philosophy towards health care. It has as its primary objective, convincing an individual to change their behaviour and adopt a healthier lifestyle. This approach is based on the premise that the expert knows best and epidemiological evidence is likely to be used to target high risk patients and health issues (for more discussion on this see Chapter 6). A health persuasion intervention is often based on the giving of information about behaviour, for example, trying to persuade a patient to undertake more exercise by outlining to them what the benefits to their health might be. This is a popular technique as it is possible for it to be relatively quick, delivered as part of a consultation and it appears to address high risk factors and individuals while offering a relatively cheap form of intervention. It also does not rely on any shift in organisational commitment to become a health promotion setting (see Chapter 10). It has been suggested that health promotion strategies in hospitals tend to rely heavily on this technique to the exclusion of other methods (Johnson and Baum, 2001).

Critics argue that if used in isolation, attempts to persuade patients to change behaviours that are expert driven and medically approved, are likely to be limited in their effectiveness (Whitehead, 2005) and point to the fact that this technique is less likely to explore whether the patient is ready or skilled enough to make changes in their lifestyle. In addition, it has been argued that the focus on the responsibility of the individual to change their behaviour does not recognise the relative powerlessness of some and the lack of choice that their situation in society may give them (Lavarack, 2005). This is because of a failure to explore the issues within the context of the patient's life and circumstances and a failure to address the wider social and economic determinants of health that we outlined in the previous chapter.

> **Case study 4.3:** Smoking cessation – brief interventions
>
> The National Institute for Health and Clinical Excellence has issued guidance on brief interventions for smoking cessation (2006) to support health care and other professionals working with patients who smoke. Brief interventions involve short five to ten minute sessions with patients and include opportunistic advice, information negotiation or referral to specialist smoking cessation services and might typically be carried out by nurses in both community and acute settings. The guidance recommends that all patients who smoke (with rare exceptions) are advised to quit and those who are not ready to quit be asked to consider the possibility and access support at a later date.

Legislative action

Legislative action is also concerned with changing behaviour but through the benevolent actions of the state or an organisation. This approach includes actions to bring about changes to national legislation, the development of national, local or organisational policies and supportive environments for health (see Chapter 10) and the provision of adequate resources to support national programmes. Such actions aim to make healthier choices easier. While interventions at this level can encourage change, universal measures are often unable to meet the specific needs of all minority groups or individuals within a population. When enforcement underpins this approach, such interventions may be met with resistance from sections of the population. A danger is that prohibitive legislation may have the effect of driving certain behaviours underground and so making it harder to access vulnerable groups and potentially increasing inequalities in health.

> **Activity**
>
> Think of legislative or regulatory action to promote healthy eating. Do you think people's behaviour should be controlled?

You may have thought of examples such as food labelling, bans on the advertising of 'junk food' during children's television viewing time or bans on vending machines in school. Whilst some may argue that what we eat should be a matter of choice, others argue that health problems such as the rising obesity epidemic demand intervention by the state.

Case study 4.4: Tobacco control

In March 2006 Scotland became the latest country to impose a ban on smoking in enclosed workspaces. The ban is intended to protect people working in pubs, clubs, restaurants and other workplaces from second-hand smoke, while also contributing to the broader aim of reducing numbers of smokers in Scotland. Penalties for breaking the ban include a £50 fine.

In England the government has made a commitment to implementing a similar policy in public places (DoH, 2004). The government outlined in its paper *Smoking Kills* (DoH, 1998), its commitment to providing services to support people giving up smoking and required each Primary Care Trust (PCT) to provide a smoking cessation service offering specialist counselling, advice and support.

A government's decision to pursue such legislative action may be directly influenced by lobbying by the public, professionals and pressure groups. Nurses can play a part in this lobbying process. The Royal College of Nursing (RCN) produced a tool kit in the run up to the 2005 General Election to encourage and support members to make their voices heard and influence political candidates. One of the key aims of their election strategy was to call for a total ban on smoking in all public places (RCN, 2005).

Community development

Community development is committed to bottom up, community-led, participatory approaches. Such interventions are based on the empowerment of communities to identify and prioritise their own needs, to work together to seek solutions to those needs and implement change as part of an ongoing process. The community involved may be a geographical community but may also be a community defined by culture, interest or social identity. Advocates argue that interventions are therefore more relevant, create a sense of ownership and are more likely therefore to be effective and sustainable. Chapter 9 discusses ways in which the nurse may work with communities.

The community development process is based on principles of social justice and equity, and requires professionals to be led by the communities they work with. This therefore becomes a potentially radical approach to health promotion which may present certain challenges for some, particularly if the priorities of the community do not match those of the professional or current health policy agenda. Community development can be a complex process that requires long-term commitment and specific resources and skills. It is also often an intersectoral approach that involves partnerships with other health agencies as well as other statutory and voluntary bodies. A nurse involved in such an approach is likely to be one among a number of key professionals undertaking work as part of a planned project and as such, involvement often requires an organisational and policy commitment. A key role for nurses within community development is in the first stages of the process (Whitehead, 2005). Effective community development begins with a process of empowerment through critical consciousness-raising whereby individuals and communities begin to question and challenge the social justice of their situation (Ledwith, 2005). Nurses have the potential to be involved in this process with both individuals and communities by raising awareness of the wider factors that determine health choices. This can then contribute to a collective action at a wider community level (Latter, 2001).

Case study 4.5: LETS Make It Better (LMIB)

Local Exchange Trading Systems (LETS) are a system of cash-free, community trading networks. Through them, members offer each other goods and services such as babysitting, gardening and decorating that can be exchanged for units. Members have accounts and can build up credit through the services they provide and can then exchange them by 'purchasing' other people's services. LMIB was set up by a community psychiatric nurse as a way of developing the scheme to involve people disabled by, or recovering from mental illness. LMIB offers members support and training so that they are confident and skilled enough to begin trading. It aims to encourage within patients a sense that they have something to contribute, to build confidence and skills while creating new relationships, to develop networks of social support and to increase access to practical services while potentially on a low income. The scheme is based on principles of involvement with the management committee being member-led.

Nurses have a role to play in schemes such as this not only through the development of initiatives but through active links and referrals into them. LMIB, for example, has developed links with hospitals and has become part of the psychiatric hospital discharge plan. The local day hospital and community mental health team have both also opened accounts with LETS (NHS Health Scotland, 2003).

Personal counselling

Interventions within this sphere are also led by, or negotiated with, the patient and are based on one-to-one work. The role of the nurse in this situation is to listen to the patient and work to empower that individual to make the changes they feel they need to make. This might involve problem solving strategies, skills development tools as well as confidence and self-esteem building. Such approaches can be used either to promote positive health and wellbeing or to prevent ill-health through disease management. Developing partnerships with patients and their family in the management of long-term conditions may be an example of such a technique. Motivational interviewing, described in Chapter 8 has also been described as a client-led change strategy.

Limitations of such an approach are the ability of individuals to sustain such changes when faced with structural social or economic issues that are beyond an individual's control but which create barriers to change.

Case study 4.6: Specialist teenage pregnancy midwife

The multi-disciplinary teenage pregnancy team at Croydon PCT includes a specialist teenage pregnancy midwife. As part of this role, the midwife works closely with some of the most vulnerable pregnant teenagers from once they are registered with the antenatal service until they are ready for the health visiting team. Through this role the midwife addresses all clinical issues but works beyond this to explore wider social, economic and emotional issues that may ultimately impact on the mother and baby's wellbeing. Support, advice and referral to other services may be given around housing, education, benefits, training, etc. Support is also given around family and relationship issues. In this way, the midwife is able to build a relationship with the young women and help develop coping strategies and skills that become important after the birth of the baby.

Each of the quadrants of the Beattie model gives rise to a different approach. Each of these four approaches can be seen to be based on a distinct set of values, objectives and political persuasions. In reality, none are likely to be effective in promoting health and reducing inequalities in health if they are adopted as the only approach. Rather, a combination of interventions is necessary. Beattie's model provides a useful framework for considering the options available when planning a project.

Activity

- Choose a health issue and identify as many interventions as you know that address this issue.
- Locate these in the appropriate quadrant of Beattie's model.
- What strengths does each of the interventions offer in addressing this issue?
- What might the limitations of each of these interventions be?
- Are most of the interventions in any one quadrant? Why do you think this is?

The role of the nurse in health promotion

The Tannahill and Beattie models, as well as other models available in the literature (Ewles and Simnett, 2003; Naidoo and Wills, 2000; Tones and Tilford, 2001) show that health promotion incorporates a broad range of activities that go beyond simple health education and lifestyle messages. The potential for nurses to be involved in all aspects of this has not been seized upon in the past and there have been calls for nurses to develop their role to include health promotion. This may involve nurses contributing to the structural development of environments that are supportive of health, encouraging participation of communities and individuals in health issues and contributing to the development of healthy public policies (Latter, 2001). While some of these activities allow the nurse to act independently and opportunistically and to become an intrinsic part of ongoing hospital work, others require the nurse to be one part of a larger, ongoing process. The latter does make it much harder for the individual nurse to see clearly how their input affects a final outcome, but is no less important.

The nurse's contribution to promoting health, whether at a direct patient level or a more strategic level, should be based on clear aims and objectives with identified goals and desired outcomes. Achieving this requires a nurse to reflect upon and be clear about the values and perspectives that underpin practice.

Summary

Health can be understood from a number of different perspectives, each of which has a different focus and results in a different approach being taken to promote health. A biomedical perspective sees health as being determined primarily by physiological risk factors and thus leads to health promotion approaches that focus on preventing disease using clinically based interventions such as immunisation programmes. A behavioural perspective focuses on the ways in which people live as being key to determining their health. Promoting health is then seen as encouraging healthier lifestyles. A socio-environmental perspective on the other hand, places emphasis on the social and economic context in which people live their lives and whilst recognising the importance of biomedical and behavioural interventions, would argue for the need for change at a more structural level. Models of health promotion are useful in scoping the field of activity and analytic models such as that of Beattie (1991) can help practitioners to interrogate their practice and be more able to justify the actions they take to promote health.

Further reading and resources

Earle S. Lloyd CE. Sidell M. and Spurr S. (Eds.) (2007) *Theory and Research in Promoting Public Health.* London, Sage.

This textbook provides a comprehensive introduction to health promotion principles and practice.

Naidoo J. and Wills J. (2000) *Health Promotion: Foundations for Practice* 2nd ed. London, Ballière Tindall.

This is a clear and accessible textbook which is easy to read and provides lots of examples of the application of theory to practice.

Scriven A. (2005) *Health Promoting Practice: the contribution of nurses and allied health professionals.* Basingstoke, Palgrave Macmillan.

A text that explores the health promotion role of numerous health care professionals with some case studies of practice.

References

Beattie A. (1991) Knowledge and control in health promotion: a test case for social policy and social theory. In Gabe J. Calnan M. and Bury M. (Eds.) *The Sociology of the Health Service.* London, Routledge.

Caraher M. (1998) Patient education and health promotion: clinical health promotion – the conceptual link, *Patient Education and Counselling,* **33**, 49–58.

Consumers' Association (2002) *Food Labels – the hidden truth.* Consumers' Association, London.

Department of Health (1998) *Smoking Kills – A White Paper on Tobacco.* The Stationery Office, London.

Department of Health (2003) *5-A-Day – general information.* Accessed online www.dh.gov.uk/PolicyAndGuidance/HealthAndSocialCareTopics/FiveADay.

Department of Health (2004) *Choosing Health: making healthy choices easier.* The Stationery Office, London.

Department of Health (2005) *The Influenza Immunisation programme – Letter from Chief Medical Officer.* Accessed online www.dh.gov.uk.

Department of Health (2006) *Screening for breast cancer in England, past and future.* Advisory Committee on Breast Cancer Screening, NHSBSP Publication no 61.

Downie RS. Tannahill C. and Tannahill A. (1996) *Health Promotion, Models and Values.* Oxford, Oxford University Press.

Ewles L. and Simnett I. (2003) *Promoting Health: A Practical Guide* 5th ed. London, Ballière Tindall.

Health Education Board for Scotland (2001) *Development of Mass Media Breast-feeding Campaign.* NHS Health Scotland, Edinburgh.

Johnson A. and Baum F. (2001) Health promoting hospitals: a typology of different organizational approaches to health promotion, *Health Promotion International,* **16**, 3, 281–7.

Katz J. Peberdy A. and Douglas J. (2000) *Promoting Health, Knowledge and Practice.* Maidenhead, Open University Press.

Latter S. (2001) The potential for health promotion in hospital nursing practice. In Scriven A. and Orme J. (Eds.) *Health Promotion: Professional Perspectives.* Basingstoke, Palgrave Macmillan.

Lavarack G. (2004) *Health Promotion Practice, Power and Empowerment.* London, Sage.

Lavarack G. (2005) *Public Health, Power, Empowerment and Professional Practice.* Basingstoke, Palgrave Macmillan.

Ledwith M. (2005) *Community Development: a critical approach.* Bristol, The Policy Press.

Naidoo J. and Wills J. (2000) *Health Promotion: Foundations for Practice* 2nd ed. London, Ballière Tindall.

Naidoo J. and Wills J. (2005) *Public Health and Health Promotion: Developing Practice.* London, Ballière Tindall.

National Institute for Health and Clinical Excellence (2006) *Brief Intervention and Referral for Smoking Cessation in Primary Care and Other Settings.* NICE London.

NHS Health Scotland (2003) *Insight: case studies in community development and health in Scotland.* NHS Health Scotland, Edinburgh.

Ontario Health Promotion Resource System *Health Promotion 101 online course.* Accessed online www.ohprs.ca/hp101/main.htm.

Royal College of Nursing (2005) *General Election Campaign Toolkit.* RCN, London.

Scriven A. (2005) *Health Promoting Practice: the contribution of nurses and allied health professionals.* Basingstoke, Palgrave Macmillan.

Tones K. and Tilford S. (2001) *Health Promotion: effectiveness, efficiency and equity* 3rd ed. Cheltenham, Nelson Thornes.

Which? (2005) *Nutritional Labelling Report.* Which? London.

Whitehead D. (2003) Incorporating socio-political health promotion activities in clinical practice, *Journal of Clinical Nursing,* **12**, 668–77.

Whitehead D. (2005) The Culture, Context and Progress of Health Promotion in Nursing. In Scriven A. (ed) *Health Promoting Practice: the contribution of nurses and allied health professionals.* Basingstoke, Palgrave Macmillan.

5

Priorities for Public Health

Jenny Husbands

Introduction

Health priorities in the UK are largely determined by morbidity and mortality data. These rates of illness and death will be influenced by factors such as socio-economic status and social factors such as age and gender, genetics, lifestyle and health behaviour as discussed in Chapter 3. The Government uses morbidity and mortality data as the basis for deciding public health priorities and for drafting legislation and policies to address these prioritised health needs. This chapter will explore some of the key public health priorities, discuss the issues behind these priorities and discuss the legislation, policies, strategies and interventions that have been devised to address public health priorities.

Learning outcomes

By the end of this chapter you will be able to:

- identify and discuss public health priorities
- discuss how public health priorities are determined
- describe how the nurse can use this information to promote health.

Public health priorities

Public health priorities can be defined as specific health and social problems that are the greatest causes of disease and death. They may become a public health concern because:

- of their impact on the health of the population as a whole
- the population are concerned about the specific health issue
- of the impact on the health budget and resources such as the National Health Service (NHS)
- health professionals and health economists may feel that these priorities can be tackled effectively by interventions, policies and legislation.

Obviously public health priorities will change over time and some may even become obsolete if, for example, the disease has been eradicated such as diphtheria, small pox and cholera due to sanitation and vaccination programmes. Conversely, some diseases and health problems have become greater public health concerns and as a result have become public health priorities, such as obesity, which has reached epidemic proportions, not just nationally but globally.

Public health priorities will also be determined and influenced by the Government's political persuasion, for example the current Government is very committed to tackling health inequalities. Previous governments have been more concerned about individual health behaviour and how that may affect the individual's health, such as smoking.

Activity

What are current public health priorities?
Why do you think the Government have chosen certain conditions
    and illnesses as public health priorities?
What do you think should be a public health priority?

Some of the current public health priorities include:

Accidents, alcohol use, cancer, coronary heart disease (CHD), diabetes, drug use, health inequalities, mental health, obesity, physical activity, sexually transmitted infections and sexual health, smoking and teenage pregnancy.

Public health priorities will be determined by research evidence, public concern about particular issues and the Government's political agenda. The Government is obviously concerned about how specific conditions and illnesses affect not only the health of the individual, but the health of the nation and more specifically the fiscal implications of managing disease and long-term conditions. As individuals, we have our own health priorities but these may be based on our own health beliefs and values and may not be supported by the evidence. As a research-based profession, it is important for the nurses to be aware of current public health priorities, policies and legislation and to work towards addressing the public health priorities as directed by policy and legislation.

In the following pages we will identify some of the current public health priorities, explore how these priorities are being addressed by public health policy and discuss the nurse's role in tackling public health priorities.

Accidents

Accidents are a major cause of morbidity and mortality for older adults and for socially disadvantaged people living in the UK. Every year 10 000 people die from accidental injury and accidents are the leading cause of death in children aged 0–14 years and put more children in hospital than any other cause. Approximately 2.8 million accidents, usually caused by falls and fires, occur in the home. Road traffic accidents account for 300 000 injuries a year and in 5% of these accidents, children are injured (DoH, 2002).

Accidents can be classified as intentional or unintentional. The former denotes injuries or accidents which were not caused by a deliberate act or omission and the latter denotes injuries which were caused by deliberate acts of violence or self-harm. Unintentional injuries include cases of suspected non-accidental injuries in children, domestic violence incidents, suicide and self-harm and elder abuse (Errington and Towner, 2005).

Accidents disproportionately affect socially disadvantaged groups. For example, deaths in residential fires affect 15 times more children from social class V (unskilled) than children from social class I (professional) and pedestrian deaths affect five times more children from social class V than children from social class I (DoH, 2002). Additionally poverty, over-crowded poor housing and a lack of social support may result in children being more at risk of accidents due to a lack of supervision or lack of safe play areas. This may be compounded by high levels of stress and an inability to purchase safety equipment which may prevent accidents from occurring (Errington and Towner, 2005).

Age is also a contributory factor in unintentional accidents as over 50% of all deaths from accidental injuries occur in adults aged 65 years and over and age-specific death and hospital admission rates increase with advancing years in women aged 65 years and over and in men aged 55 years and over. For adults aged over 65 years 85 000 serious accidental injuries and 3000 deaths were caused by falls in the UK with the most common serious injury being fractured neck of femur. For adults aged over 75 years, over 400 000 were seen in accident and emergency departments due to a fall and up to 14 000 people a year died in the UK as a result of a hip fracture (DoH, 2001b).

The Government's White Paper, *Saving Lives: Our Healthier Nation* (1998) identified accidents as a major public health priority and set targets to reduce deaths and injuries caused by accidents by October 2010. The Accidental Injury Task Force was formed in 2000 to coordinate cross-Government action and to identify appropriate evidence-based practice to prevent deaths and long-term debilitating injury from accidents. This cross-Government group incorporating departments such as the Department for Transport, Department for Trade and Industry, the Health and Safety Executive and the Office of the Deputy Prime Minister identified two specific population groups – children aged 0–14 years and adults aged 65 years and over as priorities.

Case study 5.1: The role of health professionals in domestic violence (Taket, 2003)

About one in four women will experience domestic violence at some time in their lives. Women who experience domestic violence are more likely to access health services and the health service therefore has a role to play to:

- improve availability of information on domestic violence and available services
- institute systems of enquiry about domestic violence.

Routinely enquiring about domestic violence in interactions with patients rather than selectively enquiring where there are suspicions may help to:

- uncover hidden cases
- change the perceived acceptability of violence within relationships
- make it easier for women to access support at an earlier stage
- help to maintain the safety of women experiencing domestic violence.

Nurses and other health professionals, in particular those in primary care and mental health services, are ideally placed to identify women who are experiencing domestic violence. Repeated enquiry at a number of consultations increases the likelihood of disclosure.

Activity

You are working in accident and emergency and a child aged seven years is admitted following an accident on a farm.

What is your role in accident prevention?

How could you raise the issue of accident prevention within the farming community?

Accident prevention normally involves three elements: education, enforcement and engineering. The role of the nurse in accident prevention may be at individual or population level:

- health education with patients or their carers following an accident to prevent further accidents, or minimise the injuries from this accident and appropriate first aid responses
- legislative work such as encouraging patients or carers to comply with laws and policies to try to prevent accidents from occurring, e.g. preventing accidents caused by speeding or not wearing a seat belt; wearing protective clothing; safety around moving equipment
- lobbying for changes to the environment such as fencing round domestic ponds or pools.

Cancer

Cancer is a disease process that can affect cells in any part of the body and cause them to proliferate to form a primary tumour. This primary tumour, known as a malignant tumour or neoplasm can spread and invade other cells to form metastasises (known as secondaries) which may lodge in other parts of the body and can cause a loss of function to the other cells and organs. However, some cancer cells known as benign tumours tend to grow slowly and do not invade other organs unless they are very large (Cancer Research UK, 2002).

Cancer has overtaken CHD to become the biggest single greatest cause of mortality in the UK. Every year 200 000 people are diagnosed with cancer in England and 120 000 people die from cancer (DoH, 2000a).

Figure 5.1 shows the number and incidence of cancer cases in 2004 and Box 5.1 describes some of the recent trends in cancer prevalence in the UK.

BOX 5.1 Cancer trends in the UK (DoH, 2000a)

- Numbers of newly diagnosed cases have increased with 600 new cases being diagnosed daily
- Overall mortality rates have declined
- Mortality rates for breast cancer have fallen by over 20% possibly due to better public awareness, better treatment and screening programmes
- Childhood cancers, such as leukaemia, have also seen an improvement in survival rates, with almost two-thirds of children now in remission
- Mortality rates for cervical cancer have also declined by 7% since the introduction of the cervical screening programme and better public knowledge.

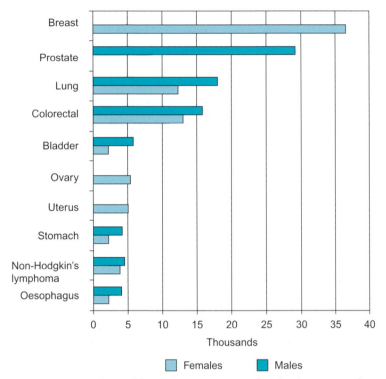

Figure 5.1 Incidence of the major cancers. Reproduced with permission from Official National Statistics, England, 2004a.

Cancer is a multifaceted issue with causes divided into the modifiable and unmodifiable. Modifiable causes include health behaviour, including a high fat diet, smoking, alcohol intake, physical inactivity, unprotected sex, being over weight and over exposure to carcinogens such as radiation. Diet plays a vital role in predisposing the individual to developing cancer; evidence has shown that a diet low in fruit and vegetables, low in fibre, high in saturated fats and high levels of alcohol consumption can predispose the individual to cancer and specifically certain forms of cancer (DoH, 1998).

Childhood nutrition could also contribute to the likelihood of developing cancer. Evidence has shown that rapid growth in childhood specifically linked to circulating levels of insulin, can predispose the child to the long-term risk of developing cancer in adult life (Davey Smith et al, 2000).

Smoking is the biggest risk factor of cancer and is closely associated with lung cancer, cervical cancer, oesophageal cancer, tracheal cancer, cancer of the larynx, stomach, pancreas and bladder. Smoking causes

---

Case study 5.2: European prospective investigation of cancer and nutrition

This is a long-term study of more than 500 000 people in ten European countries whose diet and lifestyle and health status will be followed for at least ten years. Initial findings show:

- high intakes of fibre reduce the risk of bowel cancer
- high intakes of red or processed meat increase the risk of bowel cancer and stomach cancer
- being over weight or obese increases the risk of breast cancer in women after the menopause
- being over weight or obese increases the risk of kidney or oesophageal cancer
- people with large waist circumferences or large waist to hip ratios have higher risk of pancreatic cancer
- people with the most fat in their diet had twice the risk of breast cancer
- high levels of fruit and vegetables as indicated by vitamin C levels, reduce the risk of dying early from any cause of cancer by 20%
- high intakes of milk and cheese and high levels of calcium in the diet are linked to reduced risk of bowel cancer
- high levels of fruit and vegetables do not reduce the risk of breast and prostate cancers.

Source: http://www.iarc.fr/epic/

---

approximately one fifth of all deaths which equates to 114 000 deaths per annum. Most of these are premature deaths and of the premature deaths 42 800 are from lung cancer; 30 000 are from CHD; and 29 100 are from chronic obstructive airways disease (Doll *et al*, 1994; Peto *et al*, 2003; http://www.ash.org.uk).

The incidence of most cancers reflects the social class distribution of risk behaviours. People from social class V are far more likely to smoke and therefore increase their risk of developing lung and other smoking related cancers than those from social class I (DoH, 1998). Bowel cancer is another cancer that is far more common in people from social class V than in people from social class I, possibly due to a lower consumption of fruit and vegetables by people who are socially and financially deprived. Women from social class V are also far more likely to develop cervical cancer than women from social class I (Brown *et al*, 1998). This is possibly due to lower uptakes of cervical screening, poorer access to health care services and a delay in seeking treatment (DoH, 2000a). Breast cancer, which is the most common cancer in the UK, is the exception to this patterning of disease according to social class as women from more affluent groups have a higher incidence of breast cancer possibly due to the later onset of pregnancy and breastfeeding and higher alcohol consumption (Brown *et al*, 1998).

Scenario

Mrs Mills is a 50 year old woman who has been admitted to your ward for a colostomy following a diagnosis of bowel cancer. Mrs Mills is divorced and has three children.

Mrs Mills had loose stools, distension and abdominal pain for months and eventually discussed this with the practice nurse who made an appointment with the general practitioner (GP) who referred Mrs Mills to the hospital for tests. After having a barium meal, ultrasound scan and an endoscopy, Mrs Mills was diagnosed with terminal bowel cancer.

Mrs Mills is understandably upset and angry. She feels that she has always taken care of her health and 'did all the right things', i.e. ate a healthy diet and kept her weight down and didn't smoke or drink excessively.

What would you say to Mrs Mills?

The nursing scenario above illustrates that although people may follow health advice and endeavour to live a health enhancing life, events beyond the control of the individual may impact on their health and increase their risk of developing cancer. Therefore the issues here are not about fault and control and victim blaming. Sometimes patients blame themselves for their poor health and this may add to their feelings of anger and helplessness. As a nurse, your role would be to listen, support and empathise with Mrs Mills and try to understand her feelings of anger. You could try to give Mrs Mills advice about her treatment options and encourage her to be involved in her own care planning.

So far we have considered the major causes of cancer and found that there are intrinsic factors such as genetics and extrinsic factors such as the environment in which the individual lives and works, which may increase their likelihood of developing cancer. As a result of this, it could be argued that the individual's risk of developing cancer will be determined by the type of cancer as well as other factors, some of which will be entirely outside of the individual's control. Some extrinsic factors are determined by society such as poverty and social class and again are outside of the individual's control. As a nurse, it is too simplistic and very unhelpful to blame individuals for their health damaging behaviour, e.g. if the patient smokes and subsequently develops lung cancer. Such behaviours can be because the individual feels fatalistic and unable to have any control over their lives. As a nurse, you have a pivotal role in helping your patients to take control over their lives.

The Government initiated the Cancer Plan in 2000 (DoH, 2000a) as a comprehensive strategy to tackle disease and coordinate cancer care services. This plan aims to:

- improve investment and reform service provision including increasing the numbers of doctors, nurses and allied health professions who deliver these services and providing more equipment used in the diagnosis and treatment of cancer
- reduce smoking in adults from the current rate of 28% to 24% by 2010
- reduce and address the gap between socio-economic groups in smoking rates
- reduce waiting times for diagnosis and treatment with patients having to wait no longer than a month from referral by 2005
- make a commitment to give an extra £50 million to improve access to hospice and palliative care across the country.

Nurses have an important role to play in both preventing and treating cancer. In terms of prevention, nurses can work with individuals to educate them about their risks and encourage people to lead a healthy lifestyle, e.g. stopping smoking, eating a diet high in fruit and vegetables and low in saturated fats, decreasing their level of alcohol consumption, increasing their level of physical activity and reducing their exposure to carcinogens such as radiation. This level of intervention could either target high risk groups or work with the whole population. Nurses can also work with communities to lobby for change in access and availability to health enhancing facilities, such as fruit and vegetable stalls in food drought areas or lobbying for affordable and accessible physical activity facilities.

Nurses are also involved in caring for patients on the wards or in their homes: this care could be in relation to acute care following an operation or treatment to arrest the cancer or it could be tertiary care for patients who may be terminally ill with cancer. Health promotion is often perceived to involve primary or secondary prevention (see Chapter 2) but increasingly attention is given to the management of long-term conditions. The Expert Patients Programme is run locally for different conditions and is designed to help people manage the pain, sleep problems and depression often associated with chronic conditions or terminal illness.

The role of the nurse caring for patients with cancer includes:

- having an educational role on the causes of cancer specifically in relation to health behaviours such as smoking, diet, alcohol and physical inactivity
- encouraging patients to take up preventative health services such as breast screening and cervical screening
- tackling inequalities in health as, with the exception of breast cancers, socially disadvantaged groups are disproportionately affected by cancer
- being involved in the development of policies and procedures which both address the prevention and treatment of cancer. For example nurses are involved in screening programmes such as the NHS Breast Screening Programme which employs many specialist breast care nurses to counsel, advise, support and care for women with breast cancer (DoH, 2000a).

Coronary Heart Disease (CHD)

CHD is a condition caused by blockages to the arteries by fatty, calcified deposits and a degeneration of the venous valves as a result of specific health and lifestyles behaviours, age, genetics and social class (McPherson, 2005).

- CHD is a leading cause of mortality and morbidity in the UK with 110 000 people dying every year including 41 000 people under the age of 75 years.
- For both men and women the mortality rates have declined steadily by 4% since the 1970s.
- On an international scale, the UK still has one of the highest rates of CHD and compares less favourably than the USA and Australia.
- There is a social class gradient, with men from social class I halving their CHD mortality rate since the 1970s whereas men from social class V only achieving a marginal difference. This has resulted in a steep increase in the social class gradient over the past 20 years with mortality rates for men from social class V three times higher than for those from social class I (DoH, 2000b).

Activity

What are the major health behaviours that contribute to CHD?
Are any of these health behaviours preventable?

McPherson (2005) argues that all the major risk factors are highly preventable even with patients who are at high risk due to their family history or genetics, if patients addressed their health and lifestyle behaviours, e.g. not smoking, maintaining a healthy weight, becoming more physically active, eating a low fat diet and eating five pieces of fruit and vegetables a day and drinking alcohol within recommended limits.

These factors will of course be influenced by the social circumstances in which the individual lives and will reflect the social class gradient. Smoking, for example, is far more common in social class V and amongst people between 16–44 years than in social class I. People from social class V have smoking rates of approximately 50% and as high as 60% in single parent families, whereas the smoking rate in the general population is approximately 30%. Additionally, both men and women in social classes IV and V are more likely to have high blood pressure, eat a diet low in fruit and vegetables, have poor quality housing and be in a low income occupation – all of which predisposes their risk of contracting CHD (DoH, 2000b). Figure 5.2 shows how women from lower socio-economic groups are more likely to be obese.

Minority ethnic groups, particularly Pakistanis and Bangladeshis, have a higher than average risk of developing CHD. People from these two ethnic groups living in England have premature mortality rates that are (46% for men and 51% for women) higher than the general population, and the fall in mortality rates from CHD for the general population since the 1970s had been much slower for these groups than

Percentages

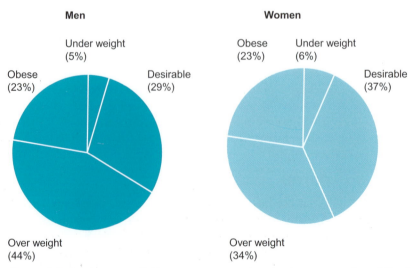

Figure 5.2 Body Mass and Obesity 2004. Reproduced with permission from Official National Statistics, England, 2004b.

for the rest of the population (Balarajan, 1996; NHS, 1996). Material deprivation as well as differences in lifestyle (see Chapter 3) may account for the differential susceptibility to CHD (Nazroo, 2001). There is some evidence that even when primary care is accessed, South Asians do not access the health care pathway early and so are more likely to be admitted as an emergency and so there are much lower rates of revascularisation. A recent report by the London Health Observatory (2006) on inequalities in access to CHD treatment, recommends effective promotion of health literacy on CHD prevention and treatment relevant to populations at high risk.

There are intrinsic factors, such as family history, which predispose an individual to CHD. Equally fetal health, which is influenced by nutrition in utero, has been found to predetermine the likelihood of developing CHD in adulthood. A low birth weight and rapid weight gain in infancy is linked with high blood pressure, insulin deficiency and resistance and a poor lipoprotein blood profile (Acheson, 1998).

Saving Lives: Our Healthier Nation (DoH, 1998) stipulated that the Government aimed to:

- reduce deaths from CHD, strokes and related disease in people under 75 years by two-fifths by 2010
- save up to 200 000 lives in total by 2010.

The immediate public health priorities identified in the CHD National Service Framework (DoH, 2000b) were to:

- introduce smoking cessation clinics
- establish 50 rapid response chest pain clinics
- reduce call-to-needle times for thrombolysis for heart attacks
- improve paramedic response times
- modernise and coordinate CHD services.

Case study 5.3: Cardiac rehabilitation

This project was initiated by a cardiac rehabilitation nurse, who worked with the User Involvement Manager and local health promotion unit to set up a rehabilitation programme for patients. The programme began in hospital where patients were given advice and invited to attend a post discharge rehabilitation programme which included exercise classes with tailored programmes of activity according to the patient's capacity and a support group which aims to maintain lifestyle changes. After the programme finished, patients were encouraged to identify changes they can sustain including health walks in the surrounding area. Such schemes

Continued

often report high adherence rates but do require ongoing monitoring and collection of data from participants usually at ten weeks, six months and thereafter annually (up to 70% of participants claim to be still leading an active lifestyle after two years).

Source: Health First (2002)

Nurses have a responsibility to assess their patients' health needs when admitting patients to wards or receiving them into their care and to plan care that takes account of their health needs, including addressing the wider influences on health; and to encourage their patients to engage in health enhancing practices such as eating a low fat/high fibre diet. Assessment should include establishing patient's diet, levels of physical activity, smoking habits, alcohol consumption and stressors (Crouch and Meurier, 2006).

Nurses have a significant part to play in CHD that could include giving opportunistic advice during other consultations or contacts in primary care or hospital admissions. Planned health promotion interventions could be during specific health education advice sessions, such as smoking cessation clinics or weight management clinics in general practice, or during out-patient clinic appointments. There are many examples of community nurses being actively involved in developing interventions such as healthy walks schemes for patients with long-term conditions such as CHD (Health First, 2002). Nurses also have a role in devising public health policies that affect health and lobbying for improvements in access and availability to health care services that relate to CHD prevention such as physical activity facilities, affordable and available healthy food, smoking and alcohol support groups.

Diabetes

Diabetes is a group of disorders which result in sustained high levels of blood glucose. The level of blood glucose is kept within a normal range by the action of insulin – a hormone secreted by the pancreas. However in diabetes, the pancreas secretion of insulin is compromised, i.e. insufficient production of insulin, a failure to produce insulin or a failure for the body to effectively utilise the insulin (insulin resistance). This high circulating blood glucose level results in a disruption of the body's ability to utilise carbohydrates and fats for energy (Hine, 2005).

Diabetes is a serious long-term condition that:

- affects approximately 3% of the population in the UK
- affects health and life expectancy, including the health of pregnant women
- has major financial and social implications for the whole population, accounting for 10% of all hospital admissions and 9% of all hospital costs
- has become more common with 1.3 million people in the UK currently living with diabetes (Hine, 2005).

There are different types and causes of diabetes:

- Type 1 diabetes usually starts in childhood or early adulthood and accounts for approximately 15% of all cases in the UK. It occurs as a result of falls in the production of insulin due to damage to the insulin producing cells in the pancreas, possibly due to a reaction in the body's immune system.
- Type 2 diabetes usually occurs in over weight middle-aged people and accounts for approximately 85% of diabetes in the population. It occurs because of the body's inability to produce enough insulin or due to insulin resistance.
- Impaired glucose tolerance and metabolic syndrome account for a proportion of those people with type 2 diabetes CHD. In this group of people central obesity, high blood pressure and abnormal blood lipids are common factors.
- Gestational diabetes occurs in a small number of pregnant women but has significant health implications such as an increased risk of spontaneous abortion, stillbirth, a higher incidence of perinatal mortality, fetal abnormalities and maternal mortality (DoH, 2001a).

Type 1 diabetes is increasing in all population groups and there has been a steep increase in the incidence in children under five years. The major risk factors for type 2 diabetes include being over weight and specifically having an apple shaped body, i.e. a centrally located fat distribution, being physically inactive and eating a high fat and high unrefined carbohydrate diet (i.e. sugar). Those most at risk are middle-aged sedentary people, but increasingly younger people are developing type 2 diabetes. In the UK type 2 diabetes disproportionately affects the South Asian, African and African-Caribbean population groups and there is a strong correlation with socio-economic status (Riste *et al*, 2001).

The National Service Framework (NSF) for Diabetes (DoH, 2001a) sets out standards for diabetes care and advocates the prevention of type 2 diabetes by:

- devising strategies to identify people who are known to have diabetes

- empowering people with diabetes to work in partnership with service providers to manage their care – this has been embodied in the Expert Patient Programme which is based on theories of empowerment, and fully engaging patients and carers
- ensuring that clinical care is of the highest standard to reduce the risk of complications developing and would include the care of children and young people with diabetes
- improving the management of diabetic emergencies including the implementation of protocols for rapid and effective treatment; this would also apply to those admitted to hospital for any reason
- improving the treatment and management of gestational diabetes (a pregnant woman with diabetes would also be subject to policy development to optimise the chance of a healthy pregnancy)
- improving the detection and management of long-term conditions (complications will be monitored and subject to review to reduce the likelihood of developing debilitating conditions and premature death).

Activity

What primary preventative health promotion advice would you give to patients on your ward in relation to the prevention of type 2 diabetes?

Primary prevention advice for diabetics should include information on healthy eating, increasing levels of physical activity, reducing alcohol intake, maintaining a normal weight, foot care and regular health checks including eye tests. Health promotion advice could also be at a secondary prevention level which targets high risk or known groups of people with diabetes. Interventions could be diabetic clinics which are facilitated by the practice nurse where practical care is given such as blood pressure monitoring, but in addition health promotion advice may be offered on how to self manage their own care. At a tertiary level, health promotion involves working with patients to enable acceptance and rehabilitation for people with complications from diabetes such as amputations, retinopathy or renal disease.

Obesity

The WHO (2000) defined obesity as a '. . . disease in which excess body fat has accumulated to such an extent that health may be adversely affected'. The incidence of obesity has increased rapidly in the last 25 years and the House of Commons Health Select Committee (2004) stated in 2004 that:

> Around two thirds of the population of England are overweight or obese. Obesity has grown by almost 400% in the last 25yrs and on present trends will soon surpass smoking as the greatest cause of premature loss of life. It will entail levels of sickness that will put enormous strains on the health service. On some predictions, today's generation of children will be the first for over a century for whom life expectancy falls.

Globally there are over one billion over weight adults and 300 million clinically obese adults. 17.6 million children under five years are over weight or obese. This has become a major contributor to chronic disease and disability. In developing countries obesity and over weight may co-exist with malnutrition and social deprivation. In Samoa 75% of the population are obese. In the Caribbean approximately 40% of women are obese. This may affect all ages and socio-economic groups but predominately it affects those who are already disadvantaged. Obesity accounts for 2–6% of total health care costs in several developed countries and in some instances as high as 7% of total health care costs (WHO, 2003). Figure 5.2 shows that about 1 : 4 men and women in England are obese.

Contributory factors to obesity include:

- an increased consumption of energy-dense nutritionally poor foods which contain high amounts of sugar and saturated fats. This may be due to a lack of awareness or a lack of choice in areas where there is a food drought
- a poor nutritional intake combined with reduced levels of physical activity will have a negative impact on the energy balance of the individual
- economic growth and subsequent increased disposable income resulting in an increased consumption of purchased foods and labour saving devices
- urbanisation which has resulted in the increased use of automated transport as the preferred means of travel
- less physically demanding work at home and in the workplace
- globalisation has resulted in greater interchange between cultures and has led to increased consumption of fast foods which combined with the other factors listed above can contribute to weight gain (WHO, 2003)

Obesity is classified as having a body mass index (BMI) of over 30 kg/m^2. This classification provides a population measurement of obesity, but there are problems with measuring weight and defining obesity in this way. For example, the mean adult BMI in Asia and Africa is 22–23 kg/m^2, whereas in North America, Europe, Latin America, North Africa and the Pacific Islands the mean BMI is 25–27 kg/m^2 (WHO, 2003). This measurement of obesity and over weight may not accurately reflect the health risk of the patient or how their weight is composed, i.e. is their weight composed of primarily muscle or fat?

Activity

How is a patient's waist circumference significant in determining their health risk?

How could a body type influence the waist circumference?

The difficulties in using a BMI as a means of calculating over weight and obesity have resulted in other forms of measurement being considered. Waist measurement has been used to determine the over weight and obese individual's risk of developing CHD and type 2 diabetes. In men, a waist measurement exceeding 37 in or 94 cm and in women 32 in or 80 cm has been offered as an alternative measurement and a means of calculating risk of developing specific diseases. Fat distribution known as apple shaped or central distribution has been found to be associated with a higher incidence of specific long-term conditions, such as CHD, breast and colon cancer and type 2 diabetes and is more common in South Asian communities, men over 40 years and post menopausal women. The WHO (2000) and the National Obesity Forum (2003) recommend that the BMI and waist circumference are used in conjunction with each other to calculate risk and assess trends.

The White Paper *Choosing Health* (DoH, 2004) prioritises obesity along with other public health priorities such as diet and physical activity but uses the BMI as its baseline. For nurses to effectively tackle obesity raises the question about definitions of obesity and the traditional way of measuring health risk versus the methods favoured by the WHO (2003). Nurses are advised to use both measurements to calculate the health risks of their patients.

Activity

Calculate your BMI (weight over height in metres^2) and measure your waist circumference.

Do these measurements take account of your gender, age, ethnicity and body type?

The National Service Framework for obesity is due to be published in 2007. The National Institute for Health and Clinical Excellence (NICE) guidelines (2004) have been developed to inform policy and interventions including the use of drugs which interfere with the body's ability to absorb fat from the diet and drugs which produce feeling of satiety in individuals. The Department of Health (2005) are developing a food and health action plan on healthy eating with a specific focus on the role of the food industry, school meals and other stakeholders in tackling obesity.

Nurses in the community will be central to the delivery of a public health agenda on obesity, for example school nurses will have a pivotal role in developing guidelines for healthy eating and promoting physical activity in schools and running weight management programmes. Hospital-based nurses will be influential in shaping the health promoting hospital (see Chapter 10) and tackling obesity through working with catering and dieticians.

Case study 5.4 illustrates a nurse initiated and nurse-led project which demonstrates the effectiveness of a multidisciplinary approach to health promotion and obesity management.

Case study 5.4: Managing obesity in the community

Be Size Wise is a nurse-led initiative which incorporates a multidisciplinary approach to obesity management and includes dieticians, physical activity instructors, primary care teams, Healthy Living Centres, Fresh Start, local businesses and other local projects such as 5-A-Day.

The project has three components to it: diet, physical activity and behaviour change and is targeted at people with a BMI of 35 or over. The exclusion criterion includes people with unstable medical conditions, people with eating disorders, pregnant women and breastfeeding mothers.

The project's aims are:

(1) to set a realistic goal for weight loss
(2) to takes on board holistic health and individual needs
(3) for a 5% weight reduction within three months and 10% within six months.

The project was evaluated for effectiveness and disclosed that in addition to a referral rate of 147 clients, an overall reduction in the following was achieved:

Waist measurement, blood cholesterol levels, blood glucose levels, joint pain, improved breathing, improved mobility, changes in eating patterns, increased participation in physical activity and improved self-esteem.

Source: Royal College of Nursing (2005)

Jeffry (2001) argues that an effective weight management programme should be more than giving patients advice on healthy eating, physical activity and monitoring, but that it should also include:

- a printed programme on weight management which includes clear dietary, physical activity and behavioural modification advice and strategies for long-term change
- suitable equipment including calibrated scales
- specified weight loss goals with energy deficits achieved through limiting energy intake and increasing energy output
- documentation of individual patient's health risks
- clearly defined follow-up procedures and regular monitoring
- other treatment options, e.g. anti-obesity drugs for appropriately selected patients.

Summary

In this chapter we have considered some of the major public health priorities in the UK and policies that have been developed to tackle these priorities. We have considered the role of the nurse and specifically in relation to the public health priorities identified.

The Department of Health (DoH, 2006) argues that nurses have a role in relation to identifying and tackling pubic health priorities and this role has been summarised as:

- tackling the causes of ill-health and not just responding to the consequences, i.e. taking on a proactive preventative health promotion role as opposed to simply treating the effects of poor health
- assessing the health needs across the population and developing programmes to address these needs rather than only responding to the needs of the individual, i.e. taking on a public health role and developing programmes of care that meet the needs of the community rather than the individual patient
- planning work on the basis of local needs, evidence and national health priorities rather than custom and practice, i.e. ensuring that action plans are evidence-based rather than based on what has been the traditional working of the ward or clinic
- working within the framework of the Local Area Agreements, i.e. ensuring that action plans are in accordance with the local areas programmes and work in partnership to share examples of good practice and resources
- using the information available about the health needs and strengths of the population to inform agreements with commissioners and local programmes of activity, i.e. ensuring that

information you use to inform practice is up to date and relevant

- multi-agency working to plan services and promote wellbeing and ensuring that you utilise local partners to deliver appropriate programmes
- identifying which groups have significant health needs and targeting resources to meet those needs
- taking action to make the healthy choices easier, e.g. giving patients all the information they need and endeavouring to make their options more accessible and available such as making sure services are at a time and venue that meets the needs of the service users
- leading or joining a multidisciplinary team rather than working alone or in opposition, i.e. making sure that you work collaboratively and cooperatively to ensure your patients receive the best available care
- influencing policies that affect health locally and nationally, i.e. ensuring that as a nurse you use your influential position to lobby for changes in care provision and policy development that affect the health of your patients
- evaluating the impact of your work, i.e. as an evidence-based profession, it is important that you evaluate the effectiveness of your work and interventions and disseminate information on good practice (DoH, 2006).

Further reading and resources

Ewles L. (Ed.) (2005) *Key Topics in Public Health: Essential Briefings on Prevention and Health Promotion*. London, Elsevier.

Key Topics is a short, easy-to-read text that provides basic information about twelve key topics in public health, such as diabetes, cancer, smoking and teenage pregnancy, and how prevention and health promotion should be tackled at community and one-to-one levels.

Action on Smoking and Health: http://www.ash.org.uk

This site provides an overview of the key tobacco facts and statistics.

European Prospective Investigation into Cancer and Nutrition: http://iarc.fr/epic/

Summary of findings from WHO/International Agency for Research on Cancer.

NHS National Institute for Health and Clinical Excellence: http://www.publichealth.nice.org.uk/

The portal for the National Institute for Health and Clinical Excellence and its public health guidance.

References

Acheson D. (1998) *Independent Inquiry into Inequalities and Health*. The Stationery Office, London.

Balarajan R. (1996) Ethnicity and Variations in Mortality from Coronary Heart Disease, *Health Trends*, **28**, 2, 45–51.

Brown A. Harding S. Bethune A. Rosato M. (1998) Incidence of health of the nation cancers by social class, *Population Trends*, **90**, 40–7.

Cancer Research UK (2002) *What is Cancer?* Accessed online http://www.cancerresearchuk.org.uk.

Crouch A. and Meurier C. (2006) *Vital Notes for Nurses: Health Assessment*. Oxford, Blackwell Publishing Ltd.

Davey Smith G. Gunnell D. Holly J. (2000) Editorial, *British Medical Journal*, **321**, 847–8.

Department of Health (1998) *Saving Lives: Our Healthier Nation*. HMSO, London.

Department of Health (2000a) *National Health Service Cancer Plan*. The Stationery Office, London.

Department of Health (2000b) *National Service Framework – Coronary Heart Disease*. The Stationery Office, London.

Department of Health (2001a) *National Service Framework – Diabetes*. The Stationery Office, London.

Department of Health (2001b) *National Service Framework – Older People*. The Stationery Office, London.

Department of Health (2002) *Preventing Accidental Injury – Priorities for Action*. The Stationery Office, London.

Department of Health (2004) *Choosing Health: making healthy choices easier*. The Stationery Office, London.

Department of Health (2005) *Food and Health Action Plan*. DoH, London.

Department of Health (2006) *School Nurse: Practice Development Resource Pack Specialist Community Public Health Nurse*. Accessed online http://www.dh.gov.uk.

Doll R. Peto R. and Whaetley K. (1994) Mortality in Relation to Smoking: 40 Years Observations on Male British Doctors, *British Medical Journal*, **309**, 901–11.

Errington G. and Towner E. (2005) Injury Prevention. In Ewles L. (Ed.) *Key Topics in Public Health: Essential Briefings on Prevention and Health Promotion*. London, Elsevier.

Health First (2002) *Executive Summary: Research Project on User Views of Kings College Hospital Cardiac Rehabilitation Service London*. Health First, London.

Hine C. (2005) Diabetes. In Ewles L. (Ed.) *Key Topics in Public Health: Essential Briefings on Prevention and Health Promotion*. London, Elsevier.

House of Commons Select Committee (2004) *Obesity*. The Stationery Office, London.

Jeffry S. (2001) The Role of the Nurse in Obesity Management, *Journal of Community Nursing,* **15**, 3. Accessed online www.jcn.co.uk/journalasp?MonthNum=03&YearNum=2001&Type=backissue&ArticleID=329.

London Health Observatory (2006) *A briefing on ethnic inequalities in access to treatments for coronary heart disease in NHS hospitals in London*. LHO, London, Elsevier.

McPherson K. (2005) Coronary Heart Disease and Stroke. In Ewles L. (Ed.) *Key Topics in Public Health: Essential Briefings on Prevention and Health Promotion*. London, Elsevier.

National Obesity Forum (2003) *Guidelines on Management of Adult Obesity and Overweight in Primary Care*. Accessed online www.nationalobesityforum.org.uk.

Nazroo J. (2001) *Ethnicity Class and Health*. Policy Studies Institute, London.

NHS Centre for Reviews and Dissemination (1996) *Ethnicity and Health: reviews of literature and guidance in the area of cardiovascular disease, mental health and haemoglobinopathies*. Report 5. University of York, NHS Centre for Reviews and Dissemination.

National Institute for Health and Clinical Excellence (2004) *Technology Appraisal No.46 The Use of Sibutramine for the Treatment of Obesity in Adults*. NICE, London.

Official National Statistics (2004a) *Cancer: 1 in 3 develop cancer during their lives*. Accessed online http://www.statistics.gov.uk/cci/nugget.asp?id=915.

Official National Statistics (2004b) *Health Related Behaviour*. Accessed online http://statistics.gov.uk/cci/nugget.asp?id=1658.

Peto R. Lopez A. and Boreham J. (2003) *Mortality from Smoking in Developed Countries 1950–2000* 2nd ed. Oxford, Oxford University Press.

Riste L. Khan F. and Cruickshank K. (2001) High Prevalence of Type 2 Diabetes in all Ethnic Groups Including Europeans in a British Inner City Relative Poverty, History, Inactivity or 21st Century Europe? *Diabetes Care,* **24**, 1377–83.

Royal College of Nursing (2005) *Be Size Wise – Weight Management*. RCN, London.

Taket A. (2003) *Tackling Domestic Violence: the role of health professionals*. Home Office, London.

World Health Organization (2000) *Obesity: Preventing and Managing the Global Epidemic*. WHO, Geneva.

World Health Organization (2003) *Controlling the Global Obesity Epidemic*. Accessed online www.who.int/nut.

Health Information and Epidemiology

Amanda Hesman

Introduction

This chapter considers how health information and epidemiological knowledge is relevant to nursing and how it can be utilised by nurses whilst caring for clients and groups of patients. Health information, including demographic and epidemiological information underpins the body of nursing theory by increasing knowledge about health. In clinical practice this knowledge includes knowing; 'who' is most likely to be affected by a disease or condition; 'why' a disease or condition is more likely to occur; 'what' steps are necessary in order to alleviate or prevent the condition and; 'how' to best care for the client or patient with that condition. Health information and epidemiology can contribute to our understanding of health by identifying the; natural history of a disease or a condition and predisposing characteristics for ill-health; best strategies to prevent ill-health and; best treatment and management of a condition. The focus is on populations and why some populations are healthier than others. Epidemiological study can also be used to orientate public services to promote health, manage chronic conditions and contribute to the evaluation of service quality. Primarily, in order to use health and epidemiological information it is necessary to be able to articulate what it is and why it is useful. Thereafter health information needs to be located and retrieved and lastly health needs to be applied to practice in order to promote health and prevent ill-health.

Learning outcomes

By the end of this chapter you will be able to:

- describe how health can be measured
- describe common sources of health information
- understand the limitations of health information
- explain frequently used epidemiological terms
- consider how epidemiological studies contribute to our understanding of health inequalities
- demonstrate how health information informs public health policy
- relate public health information accurately to your client group and translate how this information can be used to assist individuals in order to improve their health.

Health information

Demography

Demographic information includes the basic characteristics of the population and includes:

- age
- gender
- ethnicity
- mobility
- morbidity
- population growth and fertility.

This information gives a picture of the size and structure of the population, e.g. the percentage of those over 75 years. Information is also collected from the following routine data sources:

- the census of the population
- birth and abortion notifications
- disease registers
- mortality registers.

The census is coordinated from the Office for National Statistics (ONS, 2004) and provides a 'snap shot' of the resident population in the UK and occurs every ten years. The 2001 census asked for the first time a general health question with respondents being asked to assess their own health in the preceding 12 months as 'Good', 'Fairly Good' or 'Not Good'. Respondents were also asked for the first time if they had 'any long-term illness'. The data from the census is used to allocate resources

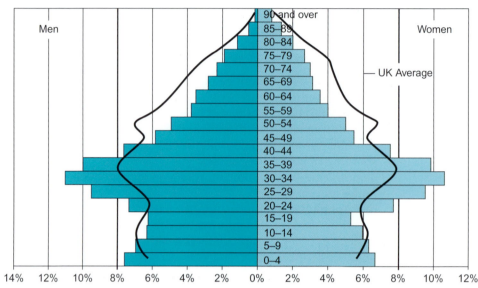

Figure 6.1 The age distribution of Lewisham, London compared to UK population 2001. (Arowobusoye N. (2004) *Lewisham Health Profile 2004.* London, PCT).

in order to plan public services including health, education and transport. Asking an individual if they have a long-term condition means that health and social services need is identified at a local level. Self reported measures of illness may not always be accurate however, as people perceive symptoms differently, some may not consider their long-term condition serious enough to report and others may over emphasise symptoms.

The population pyramid (Figure 6.1) shows the age distribution in the Lewisham population, compared to the age distribution in the UK population as at Census Day 2001 (ONS, 2001a). Compared to the rest of the UK which has 16% of the population over 65 years, Lewisham has a younger population with 11% aged 65 years and over. Information from the population pyramid can be used to plan public services appropriately.

Social classification

As we saw in Chapter 3 inequalities in health and life expectancy can be observed between groups of people from different social groups. In order to compare groups, people are placed in categories according to occupation which is meant to reflect their social status within society including their education and income. Inequalities in health can then be assessed using this information on social class together with other information on ill-health collected from disease registers and health surveys. Most ill-health demonstrates a positive social class gradient

Table 6.1 Revised social classifications.

(1)	Higher managerial and professional occupations
(2)	Lower managerial and professional occupations
(3)	Intermediate occupations
(4)	Small employers and own account workers
(5)	Lower supervisory, craft and related occupations
(6)	Employees in semi-routine occupations
(7)	Employees in routine occupations
(8)	Never worked and long-term unemployed

Source: National Statistics Socio-Economic Classification (http://www.statistics.gov.uk)

with a higher incidence in manual groups of most conditions including coronary heart disease (CHD), mental health, cancer and injuries.

The most commonly used classification to date is the Registrar General's social class classification which allocates jobs into 6 'social classes' based on occupation. The assigning of jobs to each of these bands has been criticised because dissimilar jobs have been assigned to the same group. Married women are classified by their husband's occupation which reflects a rather dated view of society. As a result a more recent classification system is now used (Table 6.1).

Deprivation measures

Inequalities in health and life expectancy are also evident between affluent and deprived geographic areas. It is possible to obtain a measure of deprivation for specific geographical areas which can then be compared with other geographical areas and importantly linked to morbidity and mortality data. Frequently used deprivation indices include, the Jarman Underprivileged Area Score, the Townsend Material Deprivation Score, the SCOTDEP index for Scotland and the Index of Multiple Deprivation for England.

The Jarman Underprivileged Area Score (Jarman, 1993) is based upon eight factors that are used to measure potential general practice work load. The Townsend Material Deprivation Score measures include unemployment (lack of material resources and insecurity), overcrowding (material living conditions), and lack of car ownership (a proxy indicator of income). SCOTDEP replaces rented housing with low social class on the grounds that the proportion of social rented housing in Scotland was sufficiently high to blunt its effectiveness as a measure of deprivation. The Index of Multiple Deprivation for England has seven domains with indicators designed to directly measure particular aspects of deprivation. The seven deprivation domains are:

- income
- employment
- health and disability
- education, skills and training
- barriers to housing and services
- crime
- living environment deprivation.

Ethnicity

The 1991 census was the first census to include a question on ethnicity with 3.3 million people describing themselves as non White. In the 2001 census the proportion of minority ethnic groups in England rose from six per cent to nine per cent – partly as a result of the addition of a category for Mixed Ethnic Groups in 2001 (ONS, 2001b). The largest proportion of this population live in London. Belonging to certain ethnic groups is associated with poorer health due to the relationship with deprivation markers such as poverty, unemployment and poor housing. The collection of ethnic data also plays an important role in monitoring access to, and uptake of, public services. Ethnicity and implicitly cultural difference will also have an effect on illness presentation, health beliefs, lifestyle and cultural practice.

Definitions and uses of epidemiology

Traditionally epidemiology studied illness in groups of people, i.e. who gets ill and why they get ill. However a contemporary definition is more inclusive: the study of the distribution and determinants of health and illness in populations. To prevent ill-health and to improve health it is necessary to identify why diseases and particular conditions occur in one population and why they do not occur in another population.

Our understanding needs to be informed by four important domains;

- the biological
- the physical environment
- the social environment
- attitudinal and behavioural factors (lifestyle).

Studying the features of a population that develop a disease or a condition, will make visible risk factors in that population that increase the likelihood of that condition developing. By studying an individual patient these risk factors remain invisible. The focus of public health enquiry is always the community or population and never the individual.

Table 6.2 Describing a population.

Biological	Physical environment	Social environment	Attitude and behaviour
• Gender • Age • Ethnicity • Genetic markers	• Rural • Green space • Transport • Access to food • Dwellings	• Social networks • Occupation • Income • Education	• Exercise • Diet • Sexual • Smoking • Alcohol • Addiction

Using the 4 domains as headings Table 6.2 lists, some 'characteristics' that could be studied in a population or community in order to identify risk factors that may be present.

Activity

The prevalence of doctor diagnosed diabetes in the population has increased in men from 2.9% in 1994 to 3.3% in 1998 and to 4.8% in 2003. Prevalence in women has increased from 1.9% to 2.5% and to 3.6% respectively (DoH, 2003).

Find out what are the many possible predispositions to diabetes using the 4 domains:

• biological
• physical environment
• social environment
• attitude and behaviour.

Associated policy that you may want to use:

DoH (2005) *Improving Diabetes Services. The NSF two years on*. DoH, London.
DoH (2001) *The National Service Framework for Diabetes*. DoH, London.

You may also wish to re-read Chapter 5 pages 78–80.

Measuring health and disease in populations

Prevalence is the total number of individuals with a disease or a condition in a defined population in a defined period of time and is usually expressed by the term 'cases'. Prevalence may be measured: at a single point in time (point prevalence); over a defined period of time (period prevalence); over an individual's entire life time (life time prevalence). Case study 6.1 uses a map to demonstrate the global prevalence of asthma and highlights some of the difficulties encountered when collecting health information.

Case study 6.1: The global prevalence of asthma

In 2001 asthma was the 25th leading cause of disability adjusted life years lost worldwide; this reflects the high prevalence and severity of asthma.

> *It is estimated that asthma accounts for about 1 in every 250 deaths world wide. Many of the deaths are preventable and are due to suboptimal long term medical care and delay in obtaining help during the final attack. (Masoli et al, 2004)*

Figure 6.2 shows data on asthma prevalence collected from the International Study of Asthma and Allergies in Childhood (ISAAC) and the European Community Respiratory Health Survey (ECRHS). This prevalence information has been collected from self reports of 'wheezing in the last 12 months' and is used to indicate the prevalence of asthma symptoms. The limitations of collecting information on asthma in this way are that self reported wheezing is not diagnostic of asthma and no single objective test to measure the frequency or severity of wheezing exists. This means that the prevalence of current asthma symptoms is not the same as the prevalence of clinical asthma. Difficulties are also encountered when comparing health information internationally as some languages do not have a colloquial term for wheezing. In an attempt to counteract this, a video questionnaire was used which showed, rather than described, the signs and symptoms of asthma. The influence of raised public and professional awareness on asthma may also impact on the reporting of symptoms making it difficult to establish the true prevalence of asthma.

The limitations that need to be considered when interpreting health information include the limitations of:

* self reporting
* definitions and interpretations of signs and symptoms
* the presence or otherwise of a single diagnostic test
* language
* increased awareness of the disease or condition.

The incidence of a disease or a condition is the number of new cases of a disease or condition that occur during a defined period in a specific population. For example, the numbers of new cases of human immunodeficiency virus (HIV) are reported in confidence to the Communi-

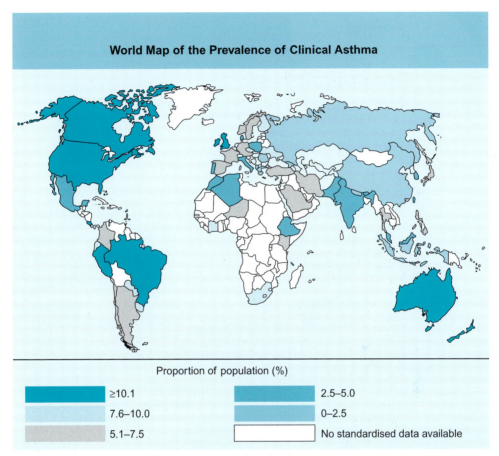

World Map of the Prevalence of Clinical Asthma

Proportion of population (%)

≥10.1	2.5–5.0
7.6–10.0	0–2.5
5.1–7.5	No standardised data available

Figure 6.2 World map of the prevalence of clinical asthma. Masoli M. Fabian A. Holt S. Beasley R. GINA Program. The global burden of asthma: executive summary of the GINA Dissemination Committee Report. *Allergy*, Blackwell Publishing Ltd.

cable Disease Surveillance Centre (CDSC) of the Health Protection Agency (HPA) each year. The incidence and prevalence of HIV has been measured since the HIV antibody test was developed in 1985. The information contained in the HIV reports to the HPA include routes of probable acquisition. The three major risk groups for HIV acquisition are: sex between men if the sexual contact is HIV positive; sex between men and women if the sexual contact is HIV positive and; injecting drug use when needles and syringes are shared with an HIV positive individual.

Activity

Figure 6.3 demonstrates the probable route of HIV infection by: year of diagnosis for the groups; sex between men; sex between men and women; injecting drug use; mother to child and; blood transfusion.

Which group has the highest and lowest prevalence of HIV?

Amongst which group has the rate of infection increased most since the year 2000?

The total number of HIV cases diagnosed in the UK up to and including those in 2004 is 71 083 (period prevalence) (The UK Collaborative group for HIV and STI Surveillance, 2005). In 1999 the number of new cases of HIV acquired heterosexually was higher than the number of new cases of HIV acquired homosexually. This means that in 1999 the incidence of HIV was higher in heterosexuals than in men who have sex with men. However, the greatest prevalence was still in the risk group of men who have sex with men. Between 1985 and 2000 intravenous drug users account for a period prevalence of 8%. In 2000 this group accounted for only 3% of the total number of new HIV cases. Although this data tells us about risk it also highlights one of the limitations of epidemiology, i.e. that it simply tells us about the scale of the problem and risk factors but not how these should be tackled as demonstrated by the sustained growth in HIV incidence.

In order for the nurse to begin to understand their role as health promoter the numbers and characteristics of people at risk of ill-health

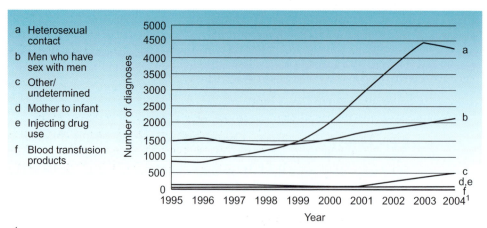

¹Numbers will rise for recent years, as further reports are received

Figure 6.3 HIV diagnoses by exposure category, UK: 1995–2004. The UK Collaborative Group for HIV and STI Surveillance. Mapping the Issues. HIV and other Sexually Transmitted Infections in the United Kingdom: 2005. London: Health Protection Agency Centre for Infections. November 2005.

or death need to be known. The most common means of measuring the health status of the population is actually by the number of people who die!

Mortality rates

Mortality data for England and Wales can be obtained from the Office for National Statistics (ONS) and in their journal the *Health Statistics Quarterly*. For Northern Ireland this information is published in the *Annual Report of the Registrar General for Northern Ireland* and for Scotland in the *Annual Report of the Registrar General for Scotland*. Not all countries have robust systems for death registration or population counting, both of which are necessary to obtain a death rate, but in the UK this information is routinely collected. All deaths must be registered by a medical practitioner within five days of the date of death. These deaths are then coded according to the International Classification of Diseases (ICD). A common problem is identifying the direct cause of death as distinct from contributory causes.

Mortality information is data that counts the number of deaths, e.g. in 2003 there were 538 254 deaths registered in England and Wales (ONS, 2005a). A number like this is not however very helpful as it does not allow any comparison across populations. To do this, we need a rate. A rate has three components:

- a numerator – the number of the population who have died
- a denominator – the total number of the people in the population
- a time period in which the deaths took place.

The crude death rate
This is the total number of deaths in a population in a year expressed as a rate per 1000 of the population and does not consider the age at which death occurred. In 1999 London's crude death rate equalled nine deaths per 1000 residents (ONS, 2005a).

The age specific death rate
This refers to deaths in an identified age group of a population expressed as a rate per 1000. In Scotland in 2003, for men and women the age specific death rate for people aged 35–44 years is 1.7 per 1000 rising to 3.9 per 1000 in those aged 45–54 years (General Register Office for Scotland, 2004).

The perinatal mortality rate
This is the number of still births and deaths within the first week of life per 1000 total births. In 2002 England and Wales had a rate of 8.3 per 1000 (ONS, 2005b) and Scotland had a rate of 8.1 per 1000 in 2004 (General Register Office for Scotland, 2005).

The infant mortality rate

This is the number of infants dead within 12 months of birth per 1000. In 2002 England and Wales had a rate of 5.3 per 1000 (ONS, 2005b) and Scotland had a rate of 4.9 per 1000 in 2004 (General Register Office for Scotland, 2005).

The cause specific death rate

This is the number of people that have died from a particular condition to the total number of cases of that condition.

Case study 6.2 demonstrates how health information from the ICD codes can be used to identify an increase in the incidence of cause specific death rate.

Case study 6.2: Using the ICD codes and death rates by cause – homicide by poisoning

This case study reveals the impact of Harold Shipman's unlawful killings on mortality statistics by cause in England and Wales. The Shipman Inquiry, an independent public enquiry set up in 2001, found that Shipman unlawfully killed 215 patients between 1975 and 1998. These killings are classified by ICD codes as 'homicides by poisoning'. As homicide, and in particular homicide by poisoning, is a rare cause of death in England and Wales these killings have a significant influence on the cause specific death rates. After the Shipman Inquiry relatives could re-register individual deaths. The case of Harold Shipman is used as a contemporary but thankfully unusual example.

Figure 6.4 demonstrates the impact that these killings by Harold Shipman had on homicide rates by comparing the original rate reported with the subsequent rate that includes the re-registered deaths.

Homicide rates for Shipman's female and male patients were greater than those for the whole of England and Wales. Between 1996–1998 Shipman's male patients had a homicide rate 610 times higher and female patients 5600 times higher than those in England and Wales.

Source: Griffiths (2003)

Epidemiological studies that utilise death rates may hope to identify specific characteristics and behaviours in that population that could be modified in order to reduce premature deaths. Descriptive studies make use of routinely collected data such as death certification data or infectious disease notification and may give a general indication into

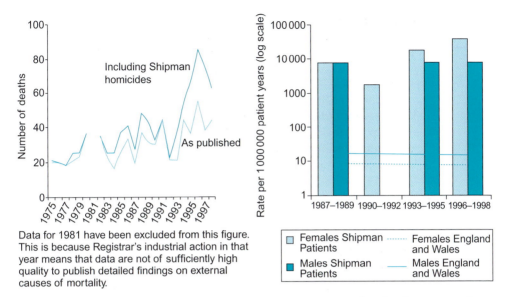

Data for 1981 have been excluded from this figure. This is because Registrar's industrial action in that year means that data are not of sufficiently high quality to publish detailed findings on external causes of mortality.

Figure 6.4 Mortality rates from unlawful killings 1975–1998. Reproduced with permission from Office National Statistics, 2003, *Health Statistics Quarterly,* **19**, 5–10.

the aetiology or cause of a disease or condition. There are categories that need to be analysed when using descriptive studies:

- when
- where
- who.

Case study 6.3: Using epidemiological data to identify cause

A Southwark energy survey in 1999 indicates that pensioners were over represented in all the indicators used to suggest fuel poverty compared to other groups. Figure 6.5 charts the number of excess winter deaths in London since 1999. Excess winter deaths are defined as the number by which deaths in the winter period December–March exceed those in the non-winter months. Generally speaking, excess winter deaths tend to increase with age and are due to CVD and respiratory disease. Low income families spend less on heating, on average indicating that they live at colder temperature levels.

Continued

Figure 6.5 indicates a downward trend in London in excess winter deaths since 1999/2000. The Southwark Healthy homes initiative provides advice on energy saving methods and grants to cover the costs of home improvements that reduce heat loss. A cold weather pack 'Beat the Cold' has been produced in partnership with local health agencies and distributed to libraries, housing centres and older people groups. The Department of Health have a 'Keep warm, keep well this winter' campaign and have produced a leaflet about fuel poverty and provide free telephone advice.

Activity

The highest perinatal mortality rate (PMR) (number of stillbirths or deaths within the first week of life) in England and Wales in 2003 by Strategic Health Authority (SHA) was in the West Midlands with 10.1 per 1000. The lowest at 6.9 per 1000 was found in both the South East and South West Health Authorities, within which the lowest rate was in Hampshire and the Isle of Wight at 6.6 per 1000 (ONS, 2003b).

Why do you think that Hampshire and the Isle of Wight have the lowest PMR mortality rate?

The following women have the lowest PMRs: women having their first child; women aged 20–29 years and; women that have a gap between their children of between 18–35 months. The PMR is higher for illegitimate births than it is for legitimate births and there is a positive social

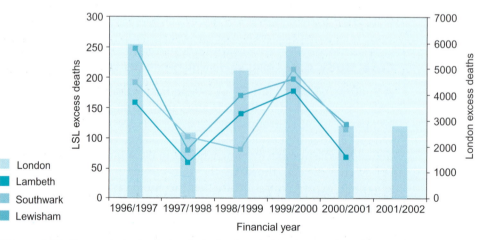

Figure 6.5 Excess winter deaths Lambeth, Southwark, Lewisham and London 1996–2002. (ONS, 2003a).

class gradient with social class V having the highest PMR. Low birth weight is correlated with perinatal mortality. Factors associated with a high PMR include: hypertension; poorly controlled diabetes; renal disease; infections that cause fetal abnormalities; severe malnutrition; smoking and alcohol (Farmer and Lawrenson, 2004).

Standardised mortality rate

The standard mortality rate is used to compare death rates between different populations. Standardisation will identify the ratio between the actual number of deaths to the expected number of deaths in a specific population. When comparing two populations that have big differences in the proportions of the very old and very young it is necessary to alter the data to take account of this difference – this alteration is known as standardisation.

In England and Wales mortality from all causes for all adults aged 15 and over has decreased in the past 40 years. The age standardised mortality rate (ASR) for all causes of death fell by over 40% in both sexes over this period. In 2001 the ASR was 821 deaths for males and 555 deaths for females per 100 000 population (ONS, 2003a).

Life expectancy

Life expectancy at birth is an estimate of the average number of years a new born baby would survive if he experienced the designated areas' age specific mortality rates for that time period throughout his life. Expectation of life at birth is used as an index of mortality and reflects both childhood and adult mortality. Differences in life expectancy are evident between countries with a high income and low income and even within countries differences can exist (Table 6.3). In countries with a low income it is not always possible to collect robust and accurate health information on life expectancy. In these countries the infant mortality rate (IMR) is often used as it is easier to collect this information. Life expectancy and infant mortality information give a proxy measure of the socio-economic status of the country, with the IMR being particularly sensitive to poverty. The population of a poorer

Table 6.3 Local authorities with the highest and lowest life expectancy at birth in the UK 2001–2003 (ONS, 2004).

Male's Life expectancy 2001–2003		Female's Life expectancy 2001–2003	
East Dorset	80.1 years	Kensington and Chelsea	84.8 years
Glasgow City	69.1 years	Glasgow City	76.4 years

Table 6.4 HALE years for females and males born in 2001 in selected European countries (WHO, 2002).

	Women	Men
Switzerland	74.4	71.1
France	73.5	69.0
UK	70.9	68.4
Poland	66.6	62.1
Latvia	64.9	55.2

country can have a shorter life expectancy and higher infant mortality rate than the population of wealthier countries.

Another way of measuring health is to measure the number of healthy years at birth that can be expected. Once we know the life expectancy and healthy life expectancy (HALE) of a population we can think about the number of years that a population will be living in ill-health or with a long-term and chronic condition. Table 6.4 lists the HALE years for females and males born in 2001 in selected European countries.

Years life lost (YLL) denotes the number of years lost due to deaths at a premature age. To calculate this it is assumed that everyone may live to some arbitrarily chosen age based on life expectancy, and that death at a younger age means that some future life years have been lost. When reading research papers that use YLL as a marker of ill-health it is important to know the chosen age of life expectancy for that population.

Morbidity

Mortality data alone does not adequately represent the health or ill-health of the population. Morbidity data measures the psychological and physical health illness and disability experienced by a population. Chronic conditions such as degenerative joint diseases like arthritis and mental health illnesses like depression may not be the primary cause of death but can cause severe disability. Morbidity data can be used to describe the experience and impact that a health problem may have and measures the burden of a disease or condition. Other methods that measure the burden of disease include 'disability-free life expectancy' and 'disability adjusted life years' (DALYs). DALYs combine years of life lost from premature death with loss of healthy life from disability. Premature death is the difference between the age at death and life expectancy at that age in a population with a low mortality.

Activity

This WHO (2002) tells us that the percentage of the global total of individual DALYs are as follows:

- infectious and parasitic diseases – 24.5%, of which HIV acquired immune deficiency syndrome (AIDS) accounts for 6% and diarrhoeal diseases 4.3%
- respiratory infections – 6.4%
- nutritional deficiencies – 2.2%
- malignant neoplasms – 5.2%, of which trachea, bronchus and lung cancers account for 0.8% and breast cancer 0.4%.

Why do you think that diarrhoeal diseases cause greater ill-health than breast cancer?

Using the Public Health Observatory that covers your region and the Health Protection Agency try to find the health information related to food borne illness and cancer.

How many cases of food poisoning were reported for a 12 month period?
How many new cases of lung cancer and breast cancer were diagnosed?
What possible reasons are there for more cases of lung cancer to be diagnosed than breast cancer?

The above information informs us that at a global level in 2001 the burden of disease from diarrhoeal disease (4.3%) is far greater than the burden of disease from breast cancer (0.4%). If we compare lung cancer with breast cancer there are 100% more DALYs attributable to lung cancer than breast cancer due to the fact that the vast majority of breast cancer is diagnosed in women.

Surveillance of health and the collection of health information

There are two distinct types of surveillance: surveillance to assess acute health trends such as communicable diseases, which shall be explored in greater detail in Chapter 7, and surveillance of longer health trends which are assessed with the use of disease registers. There is a wide diversity of data collected which can provide us with a large amount of information about the population. Some examples are given in Box 6.1.

BOX 6.1 Sources of data and health information

Routine registration and notification (birth, death, marriage)
Cancer registry
Communicable diseases
International Classification of Disease (ICD)
National Health Service (NHS) statistics (waiting lists, length of
    bed stay, completed consultant episodes)
Service uptake and utilisation
Census
Measures of deprivation
Health and disease scales
Quality of life surveys
General household survey
Social information (benefit levels, crime statistics, unemployment,
    class classification)
Smoking and food surveys.

Activity

Find out some statistics about your local area.
    What are the main causes of death? What is the standardised
mortality rate (SMR) of the population of the electoral ward that
that you live in?
    Find out what the index of multiple deprivation or similar depri-
vation index is for your area?

Electronic resources that you will need to use to answer the above
question include:
www.gro-scotland.gov.uk/statistics/library
www.nisra.gov.uk
http://neighbourhood.statistics.gov.uk/dissemination/

Mortality from all causes is a good indicator of the general death rate.
When using SMRs as a measurement, deaths below the age of 75 years
are deemed premature based on the assumption that this is average
life expectancy. For some diseases, such as female breast cancer, there
is the potential for health care service to prevent almost all deaths, at
least within certain age groups and so such deaths, suicide and road
traffic deaths, for example, may be considered preventable through
public health policies, wider social interventions, or a combination of
these.

    There are several reasons for health information being incomplete
in a population, ranging from an 'unwell' person feeling healthy and
therefore not presenting at their general practitioner (GP) practice to

poor service orientation that deters presentation. The accurate recording of health information relies on the following:

- an 'unwell' person presenting to a GP surgery
- the GP making a correct presumptive diagnosis
- the GP requesting the correct investigations
- the accuracy of the test result also called 'positive predictive value'
- the documentation of the correct diagnosis in the patient's notes which is normally done by using ICD10 classification code
- the entry of that code into appropriate health database

Many conditions are under reported and so a proportion of the
population may be ill but not seeking help. Morbidity data from those
receiving or awaiting care thus represent just the tip of the iceberg.

Activity

List the possible reasons why an 'unwell' person may not see their
GP.

Research into the experiences of men and women with CHD by Tod
et al (2001) identified six categories that hinder full use of primary and
secondary health services: structural factors; personal factors; social
and cultural factors; past experiences and expectations; diagnostic
confusion and knowledge and; awareness. Delay, denial and self-
management by individuals means that the full extent of symptoms
often remained hidden from GPs. It is also known that more women
remain underrepresented and undiagnosed with CHD when compared with men.

The role of the nurse in using health information

In order to be able to promote the health of patients and clients and
contribute to preventing further ill-health, the nurse needs to understand how common the condition is and what the risk factors for a
condition or disease are. Epidemiological studies highlight risk factors,
for example we know that elderly people from nursing homes with
repeated hospital admissions are likely to have methicillin-resistant
Staphylococcus aureus (MRSA) cultured. For the nurse, epidemiological
studies may also show what information the nurse may need to decide
appropriate intervention, for example we know that referral to a community exercise programme sustains longer change in physical activity
when compared with written information and brief advice from a
health professional. To enable the nurse to practice evidence-based

nursing the following skills need to be developed: seeking information; appraising information; extracting findings; synthesising information and; applying this new information to the clinical context. Because knowledge is constantly changing and developing the nurse needs to remain up to date. To assist the nurse to remain contemporaneous in knowledge the following should be used to inform evidence-based practice:

- treatment guidelines and protocols
- integrated care pathways (ICPs)
- patient group directives (PGDs)
- the National Institute for Clinical Excellence (NICE).

Every student should have access to electronic sources of information such as the National Electronic Library for Health (NELH) (a gateway to a virtual health library) and the Cochrane Library. Electronic databases such as CINAHL and Medline readily provide the means for a comprehensive literature search. In order to use electronic sources of information nurses will need retrieval skills and have a good knowledge of information technology.

Scenario

You are a nurse caring for someone with CHD.
   How would you answer the following questions?

- Did my drinking alcohol make me have this?
- My father died of angina at 55 years – could that have something to do with it?
- I am very unhappy in my job – can stress make me worse?
- What can I do to make myself better?
- When can I have sex again?
- What is the best way to lose weight?

As a nurse you need to know:

- What are the risk factors for CHD?
- Which lifestyle behaviours can precipitate CHD?
- What is the impact of poverty on health behaviour?
- The effectiveness of brief interventions for alcohol dependence.
- What tools there are to assess alcohol dependence.
- What support is available to help people reduce over consumption of alcohol and food.
- How cardiac rehabilitation programmes can encourage and maintain recovery.

Summary

This chapter has demonstrated how epidemiology and health information can be used to describe populations and their health and assist the nurse in understanding how the individual is part of a bigger picture. Knowing and being able to apply the 'when', 'where' and 'who' alerts the nurse to consider potential threats to health and wellbeing for the individual and should inform nursing practice. Challenges for the nurse include understanding frequently used epidemiological terms and understanding how population-based information is relevant to care delivery. Additionally, the nurse needs to be able to identify the necessary health information to be able to deliver effective and efficient nursing care – this nursing care may be therapeutic, palliative or preventative. In order to do this the nurse needs to know how and to have the information technology skills to access relevant health information from credible sources.

Further reading and resources

Health profiles can be used by local authorities and the health service to highlight the health issues for their local authority area and to compare them with other areas. The profiles are designed to show where there are important problems with health or health inequalities. They can be accessed from the Association of Public Health Observatories at http://www.apho.org.uk.

There are many accessible textbooks providing introductions to epidemiology. The following chapters provide shorter overviews and examples of how the nurse can use health information:

Katz J. (2002) Studying populations. In Katz J. Peberdy A. and Douglas J. (Eds.) *Promoting Health Knowledge and Practice* 2nd ed. Buckingham, Open University.

Mason T. and Whitehead E. (2003) *Thinking Nursing* Buckingham, Open University.

Mulhall A. (2001) Epidemiology. In Naidoo J. and Wills J. (Eds.) *Health Studies and Introduction*. Basingstoke, Palgrave Macmillan.

Association of Public Health Observatories: http://www.apho.org.uk.

General Register Office for Scotland: http://www.gro-scotland.gov.uk/statistics/library.

National Institute for Clinical Excellence: http://www.publichealth.nice.org.uk.

National Statistics/Neighbourhood Statistics: http://www.neighbourhood.statistics.gov.uk/dissemination.

Northern Ireland Statistics and Research Area: http://www.nisro.gov.uk.

Office for National Statistics: http://www.statistics.gov.uk.

World Health Organization: http://www.who.int/en/.

References

Arowobusoye N. (2004) *Lewisham Health Profile 2004.* London, Lewisham PCT.

Department of Health (2001) *The National Service Framework for Diabetes.* DoH, London.

Department of Health (2003) *Health Survey for England.* DoH, London.

Department of Health (2005) *Improving Diabetes Services. The NSF two years on.* DoH, London.

Farmer R. and Lawrenson R. (2004) *Epidemiology and Public Health Medicine.* Oxford, Blackwell Science.

General Register Office for Scotland (2004) *Table 5.1 Death rates by sex and age Scotland 1946 to 2003.* Accessed online http://www.gro-scotland.gov.uk/files/04t5-1.pdf.

General Register Office for Scotland (2005) *Table 4.2 Stillbirth, perinatal, postneonatal and death rates, Scotland 1946 to 2004.* Accessed online http://www.gro-scotland.gov.uk/files/04t4-2.xls.

Griffiths C. (2003) The Impact of Harold Shipman's unlawful killings on mortality statistics by cause in England and Wales, *Health Statistics Quarterly,* **19**, 5–10.

Jarman B. (1993) Identification of underprivileged areas, *BMJ,* **286**, 1705–9.

Masoli M. Fabian D. Holt S. Beasley R. and GINA Program (2004) The global burden of asthma: executive summary of the GINA Dissemination Committee Report, *Allergy,* **595**, 469–78.

Office for National Statistics (2001a) *Census 2001 – ethnicity and religion in England and Wales.* Accessed online http://www.statistics.gov.uk/census2001/profiles/commentaries/ethnicity.asp.

Office for National Statistics (2001b) *Census 2001: the most comprehensive survey of the UK population.* Accessed online http://www.statistics.gov.uk/census2001/census2001.asp.

Office for National Statistics (2003a) *Annual Public Health Report: Excess winter deaths: Lambeth, Southwark, Lewisham and London 1996–2002.* ONS, Southwark.

Office for National Statistics (2003b) *Table 2 Births, perinatal and infant mortality statistics 2003.* Accessed online http://www.statistics.gov.uk/StatBase/Expodata/Spreadsheets/D8518.xls.

Office for National Statistics (2004) *Geographic inequalities in life expectancy persist across the United Kingdom.* Office for National Statistics, London.

Office for National Statistics (2005a) *2003 Mortality statistics: cause, England and Wales.* Accessed online http://www.statistics.gov.uk/downloads/theme_health/HSQ25.pdf.

Office for National Statistics (2005b) *Infant and perinatal mortality by social and biological factors, 2004.* Accessed online http://www.statistics.gov.uk/downloads/theme_health/HSQ28.pdf.

Tod D. Read C. Lacey A. and Abbot J. (2001) Barriers to uptake of services for coronary heart disease: qualitative study, *British Medical Journal,* **323**, 1–6.

The UK Collaborative Group for HIV and STI Surveillance (2005) *Mapping the Issues. HIV and other Sexually Transmitted Infections in the United Kingdom: 2005.* Health Protection Agency Centre for Infections, London.

World Health Organization (2002) *The World Health Report 2002: Reducing Risks, Promoting Healthy Life.* WHO, Geneva.

Protecting the Health of the Population

Amanda Hesman

Introduction

Health can be 'protected' by preventing disease and illness and be 'promoted' by supporting and maintaining a healthier lifestyle. This chapter will focus on the former and introduce the nurse to the concept of health protection and explore the methods used to safeguard the population's health. In Chapter 6 the importance of health information and epidemiology was explored and we shall now demonstrate how this data can be used to prevent ill-health by informing population strategies that protect health. This chapter will demonstrate how the public's health can be protected through population strategies such as screening and immunisation. Within this contemporary context of screening, active immunisation and better treatment of acute infections, the shifting pattern of disease and ill-health from communicable to non-communicable diseases will be described together with a discussion of current public health threats. The responsibility of the National Health Service (NHS) and its public health function will be discussed in relation to its duty for surveillance and the management of incidents and outbreaks.

Learning outcomes

By the end of this chapter you will be able to:

- demonstrate knowledge of the principles of population-based screening programmes
- demonstrate knowledge of the principles of vaccination programmes
- describe the principles of surveillance, prevention and control of infectious and communicable diseases
- understand the nurse's role in communicating 'risk'

The changing pattern of disease and ill-health

The communicable disease epidemics of nineteenth century England
– diphtheria, typhus, cholera and tuberculosis began to be controlled
with the introduction of sanitary reform including the provision of
clean water and safer disposal of sewage. In the twentieth century with
the development of vaccination programmes and antibiotic therapy
this decline in mortality was progressed even further although outbreaks, e.g. influenza can still occur. With a reduction in absolute
poverty and an improvement in nutrition and sanitation there has been
a reduction in the prevalence of communicable disease and a corresponding increase in prevalence of non-communicable disease. Non-
communicable disease can include coronary heart disease (CHD),
diabetes, osteoarthritis, chronic pain, alcoholism and mental illness.
Many non-communicable diseases are preventable and treatable but
only in the early stages of development. Whatever proves to be the
impact of screening in the control of non-communicable disease, the
incidence and prevalence of non-communicable diseases such as
cancer and chronic ill-health will only increase with increased life
expectancy.

Globally and nationally the public health picture is quite diverse,
with health issues including known 'emerging' and 're-emerging
threats'. The term 'emerging' refers to newly identified and previously
unknown infectious agents that will or have the potential to cause a
public health problem. Over the past 30 years 30 new diseases have
emerged. The term 're-emerging' refers to infectious agents that are
known with a previously low prevalence but are now causing a public
health problem.

Current public health threats include:

* known diseases, such as malaria and tuberculosis cause high mortality and morbidity in continents such as Africa and Asia which
  the Global Health Fund is combating with the 'Roll back malaria'
  and 'Stop TB initiative' programmes
* newly identified diseases include the hepatitis C virus which was
  first identified in 1989 and the first cases of variant Creutzfeldt-
  Jakob disease (vCJD) (a transmissible spongiform encephalitis from
  cattle) was identified in humans in the UK in 1996
* Human immunodeficiency virus/acquired immune deficiency
  syndrome (HIV/AIDS) was first recognised in 1981. In some African
  countries one in four of the living population have HIV/AIDS
  and when co-infection occurs with tuberculosis (TB) mortality
  increases
* the re-emergence of old diseases in the UK, e.g., the declining trend
  in TB has been reversed

- the emergence of CHD as a leading cause of death in poor countries
- individual resistance to micro bacterial drugs due to poor prescribing and poor adherence
- mutation and modification of the genetic composition of bacteria and viruses such as HIV and gonorrhoea in order to survive adverse conditions such as antibiotic and viral therapy
- with increased global travel, population migration and the import and export of food products, disease can travel and 'developing' world viruses can be found in the 'developed' world. For example in 1999 West Nile Virus was identified for the first time in New York although it had previously only been found in Africa, Asia and Eastern Europe
- global epidemics known as pandemics. Experts predict a pandemic of influenza due to the emergence of a new flu virus A/H5N1 (avian influenza)
- the increased potential for the deliberate release of biological and chemical agents. This took place on the Tokyo underground in March 1995 with the release of the nerve gas sarin
- natural disasters such as the Tsunami in December 2004
- manmade disasters such as the Chernobyl nuclear explosion in 1996.

Protecting populations: the 'bigger picture'

Public health policy has benefit for the population and not just the individual and it is this principle that underpins population screening and vaccination programmes. Health protection is a collective good because the majority of the population will benefit rather than the individual. This raises ethical issues – for example specific patient consent is not required for public health surveillance programmes that aim to establish prevalence of communicable diseases if samples are anonymous (HPA, 2004).

Public health is to do with the health of populations and in order to protect and improve the health and wellbeing of populations, collective action is necessary. This collective action can be mediated by public health regulation. In order to protect the health of populations it is necessary for public health policy to provide for:

- surveillance, e.g. of immunisation uptake and antenatal screening
- notification, e.g. of communicable diseases such as TB and measles
- regulation, e.g. of NHS microbiology laboratories and food standards
- jurisdiction, e.g. the protection of confidentiality to do with sexually transmitted infections by The NHS (Venereal Diseases)

Regulations 1974 and port control that prohibits the movement of animals unvaccinated against rabies into the UK.

Vaccination

Vaccinations fall into the category of primary prevention as they aim to prevent the onset of infectious disease that can have serious consequence. Vaccination programmes intend to give lasting active immunity against infection and in the UK there are comprehensive vaccination programmes for:

- diphtheria, tetanus, pertussis, polio, Hib, (DTap/IPV/Hib), given at two, three and four months
- measles, mumps, rubella, (MMR) given at 12–15 months
- seasonal influenza recommended for at-risk groups and those aged over 65 years
- pneumoccocal infection recommended for at-risk groups and those aged over 65 years

These vaccination programmes have significantly reduced mortality and morbidity. Herd immunity is the term given to the resistance of groups of people to infection and is dependent upon the percentage of the population that have been vaccinated. To be effective, herd immunity does not necessarily require 100% of the population to be vaccinated because susceptible people in the population will be shielded from exposure to infected people by immune people in the group. In order to obtain herd immunity for measles the percentage of the population that require vaccination is 90%.

There has been an assumption that everyone would take advantage of a free vaccination service. However, parents' lack of experience of past common-place diseases, such as measles, lessens their fears of the disease itself and replaces it with a fear of the vaccination. This has resulted in a sub-optimal uptake in some populations. As a result measles outbreaks have occurred in school children. Some research may indicate that it has been difficult for a parent to make an informed choice as health professionals tend to emphasise the benefits of vaccination with little information being given on the risks (Lewendon, 2002).

The following groups are also at risk of low uptake of immunisation (DoH, 2005):

- children in care
- young people who missed previous immunisations
- children with physical or learning difficulties
- children of lone parents
- children not registered with a general practitioner (GP)

- children in larger families
- children who are hospitalised
- minority ethnic groups
- vulnerable adults such as asylum seekers and the homeless.

This inequality in immunisation uptake may be due to barriers to accessing health services.

Activity

Patient advocacy is concerned with providing active support for the patient and most nurses will have been taught that advocacy is a central tenet of nursing. But what happens when the patient's wishes are in conflict with recommended good practice and the behaviour of one individual impacts upon the remainder of the population?

   What do these tensions mean for your practice as a nurse?

   What should you do in these situations?

   Should you use persuasive communication to get patients to follow recommended practice, e.g. should health visitors persuade a new parent to have their infant vaccinated?

There is a philosophical tension between doing good for the population, e.g. promoting a screening test or vaccination and acting in a paternalistic manner. At one level advocacy relates to the concept of informed consent in which the health professional provides information for the individual for them to make a decision. There are inherent power imbalances in the patient/nurse relationship and one way that nurses can use this power is by persuasion (Cribb and Duncan, 2002). Therefore advocacy can be seen as a refined manipulative strategy that ensures that the patient complies with health care requests. Indeed even the UK Public Health Association (2005) recognises that there is little role for choice in public health – 'Public health is principally about organising society for the good of the population's health: at this level of concern, it is no more a matter of individual choice than the weather'.

Screening

Screening programmes fall into the category of secondary prevention as they aim to halt the development of disease. Population screening programmes should contribute to the reduction of disease and disability by identifying those at an early stage of disease progression when treatment is beneficial. Understandably many people will only seek medical advice with the onset of signs and symptoms. Screening aims to identify those individuals that have developed disease pathology before the onset of obvious symptoms.

Screening has been defined as 'a public health service in which members of a defined population, who do not necessarily perceive they are at risk of, or are already affected by a disease or its complications, are asked a question or offered a test, to identify those individuals who are more likely to be helped than harmed by further tests or treatment to reduce the risk of a disease or its complications' (www.nsc.nhs.uk).

There are various approaches to population screening:

Selective screening

This is when screening is restricted to identifiable groups identified by behaviour or risk, e.g. hepatitis C screening of intravenous drug users (IVDU). The aim of selective screening is to identify a specific disease or predisposing condition in those with a known risk factor.

Mass screening

This is when everyone is invited, regardless of risk, to attend for testing in a systematic programme which covers the whole population over a defined period of time, e.g. cervical screening. The aim is to test large numbers of people for a predisposing condition without specific regard to their individual risk factors for having or developing a condition or disease.

Anonymous screening

This is when screening is carried out without the individual's knowledge in order to establish the prevalence of a disease or condition in a given population. For example the Anonymous Prevalence Monitoring Programme (UAPMP) that commenced in 1990 aims to measure the distribution of unrecognised (undiagnosed) infection and associated risk factors for HIV, hepatitis B and hepatitis C.

Routine screening

This is when screening is carried out pre- and postnatal and throughout childhood. For example prenatal screening can be used to assess risk and assist in informed decision regarding the continuation of the pregnancy and to help prepare psychologically for any physical and mental limitations that the infant may have.

Genetic testing

This is when screening is carried out to identify individuals at risk of an inheritable condition. Although not strictly speaking population-based screening, genetic screening does have major implications for some groups, such as Ashkenazi Jews amongst whom 1 in 25 carry Tay-Sachs – genetic disease that develops progressive neurodegeneration (Kirk, 2005).

Screening can also be opportunistic by offering a screening test for an unsuspected disorder at a time when a person presents to the doctor for another reason. Opportunistic screening can be used as a strategy to maximise participation rates in mass and selective screening programmes. All nurses having made an assessment of need, have the opportunity to ask patients if they have participated in a relevant screening programme and if not, explore their concerns regarding the test. A screening test in itself does not reduce the risk or prevent ill-health. Screening tests look for signs of possible problems and help identify individuals who have an increased risk of having or developing a health related problem. Not all screening tests are diagnostic, for example a nuchal translucency scan, taken between 11 and 13 weeks of pregnancy, measures the risk that the baby has Down's syndrome. The diagnostic test offered to confirm the presence of Down's syndrome is called chorionic villus sampling.

Any screening test with the intention of screening a population needs to be evaluated for efficacy as part of a screening programme. To appraise the viability, effectiveness and appropriateness of a screening programme, the condition, the test, the treatment and the screening programme itself need to be scrutinised. The UK National Screening Committee (2000) has adapted Wilson and Junger's classic criteria for evaluation and includes the following:

The condition
- The condition should be an important health problem.
- All cost effective primary prevention interventions should be implemented as far as practical.
- The epidemiology and natural history of the condition needs to be understood with a detectable risk factor or disease marker and a latent period or early symptomatic stage.

The test
- The test should be acceptable to the population.
- There should be an agreed policy on the further diagnostic investigation of individuals with a positive test result and on the choices available to those individuals.
- There should be a simple, safe, precise and validated screening test. The two measures that describe the validity of a screening test include sensitivity and specificity:
  - sensitivity is the proportion of people that have the disease and have a positive result. A test that is very sensitive will give a high proportion of false positives

— specificity is the proportion of people that are free from the disease and have a negative result. A test that is very specific will give a high proportion of false negatives.

The treatment

- There should be agreed evidence-based policies covering which individuals should be offered treatment and the appropriate treatment to be offered.
- There should be effective treatment or intervention for patients identified through early detection, with evidence of early treatment leading to better outcomes than late treatment.

The screening programme

- There is evidence from randomised controlled trials that the screening programme reduces mortality and morbidity. For screening programmes that aim to give 'informed choice' there must be evidence that the test accurately measures risk.
- The screening programme is clinically, socially and ethically acceptable to the public and health professionals.
- The benefit from the screening programme should outweigh the physical and psychological harm.
- The screening programme needs to offer value for money.

Activity

If you were to apply the Wilson and Junger's classic criteria would you recommend a national screening programme for:

- asthma
- depression
- bowel cancer?

Asthma would not be recommended for a national screening programme as there is not a phase in which early detection would lead to a better outcome with treatment. Additionally, once symptoms are apparent, asthma can be readily diagnosed on clinical examination and be adequately managed. Depression would not be recommended as there is no validated test or assessment for depression at a population level and there is no reliable demarcation of depression from social and situational unhappiness (Summerfield, 2006). Current guidelines (NICE, 2004) do not recommend anti-depressants as the primary intervention for mild/moderate depression which account for the majority of cases. Furthermore, it is most likely that a national screening programme would not be socially acceptable. The potential for a national screening programme for bowel cancer has been debated widely in terms of acceptability and effectiveness. The outcome of a pilot screening programme (DoH, 2003) has resulted in a national screening programme for bowel cancer commencing in 2006 for men and women aged 60–69 years. This age group has been identified as the group most likely to benefit because eight out of ten people who develop bowel cancer are over 60 years.

Despite rigorous criteria, screening is not foolproof. False positive results can give rise to unnecessary and painful investigations such as biopsies, increase psychological morbidity with needless anxiety and deter future programme participation. False negative results will give false reassurance of being disease free and if symptoms do develop, may deter individuals from seeking medical advice. Additionally national screening programmes are more effective at detecting slow growing cancers as opposed to the more aggressive types of cancer that can progress rapidly in between screening tests.

Activity

What knowledge does the nurse need to have in order to understand the concepts of sensitivity and specificity and how can this information be best conveyed to the patient concerned?

The best way to convey this information is as part of a pre-test discussion in order to obtain informed consent. Within this pre-test discussion an explanation of the possible result should be given be it negative, positive, seen, not seen or inconclusive. The nurse also needs to know how to interpret the result and the likelihood of the result being true. For example a woman recalled for a repeat cervical cytology may be concerned that she has invasive carcinoma, when in fact her result indicates mild dysplasia (CIN1) which in all probability will resolve without intervention.

- The nurse needs to understand whether the screening test is diagnostic or not, and will need to make an assessment of the woman's understanding. For example, mammographies do not give a diagnosis and are very sensitive; this results in a high number of false positives that require invasive investigation for an accurate diagnosis to be made.
- The nurse needs to be able to make a judgement as to how and to what extent to best communicate this information.
- The nurse needs to know the recommended procedure for establishing a definitive diagnosis.

Population screening programmes require a high level of participation for three reasons:

(1)   to be cost effective
(2)   to ensure adequate evaluation
(3)   to reduce levels of morbidity and mortality.

It is important to consider those populations and groups of people that are less likely to participate in population screening programmes and what measures can be taken to rectify the situation. For example, those not registered with a GP such as travellers, those from a lower socio-economic group, those that are deaf and those with an intellectual impairment are less likely to participate. It is also significant that individuals from the highest risk groups have the highest non participation rates. For example, those women that are at more risk of developing cervical cancer are those less likely to attend to be screened. The poor response of high risk groups severely compromises the effectiveness of any screening programme.

Activity

In addition to a person with Down's syndrome being included in national screening programmes, good practice recommends that they also participate in selective screening at different stages in their life.

What additional screening tests does this entail?

The following additional screening tests are recommended for an adult with Down's syndrome:

- thyroid function tests for hypothyroidism
- eye and hearing tests for cataracts, keratoconus and sensorineucral hearing loss
- tests for dementia due to an association between Down's and Alzheimer's. Having an extra chromosome 21 gives a higher chance of developing neuropathological changes of Alzheimer's disease.

The UK has several national screening programmes and the UK National Screening Commitee regularly reviews whether evidence supports the introduction of new screening including aortic aneurysms, osteoporosis, cardiomyopathy, ovarian cancer and syphilis. Table 7.1 shows the current national screening programmes.

Table 7.1 Current national screening programmes.

Name of screening test	Diagnostic	Type of screening	Population
Mammography	No	Mass	Women aged 50–70 years
Cervical screening	No	Mass	Women aged 20–64 years
Hepatitis B	Yes	Selective	Health Care Workers (HCW) Men that have sex with men IVDUs (intravenous drug users) Sexual contacts of those with infectious hepatitis B virus (HBV)
Antenatal HIV	Yes	Mass	All pregnant women
Bowel cancer	No	Selective	All men and women aged 60–69 years
Chlamydia	Yes	Selective	Men and women aged under 25 years
Diabetic retinopathy	Yes	Selective	Diabetics

Surveillance, prevention and control of communicable diseases

United Kingdom

The Health Protection Agency (HPA) was established in April 2005 with three separate centres that are responsible for the protection of the public health of the UK:

- the Centre for Infections
- the Centre for Radiation, Chemical and Environmental Hazards
- the Centre for Emergency Preparedness and Response.

The HPA Centre for Infections is responsible for the surveillance of infectious diseases, providing specialist microbiology reference services, detailed epidemiological information and coordinating investigations into epidemics and outbreaks of infections.

The surveillance of a communicable disease is a fundamental activity required for an effective disease prevention and control programme. Surveillance is used to:

- estimate the size of a health problem
- detect outbreaks of an infectious disease
- characterise disease trends
- evaluate interventions and prevention programmes
- assist with health planning
- identify research needs.

In the UK a network of Public Health Observatories (PHOs) exist. In England nine were established in 2000 with each PHO identifying regional priorities and taking specific national leads. Each PHO monitors health and disease trends and works in partnership with local statutory and non statutory agencies in addressing health inequalities.

Activity

Figure 7.1 illustrates the prevalence of chlamydia in the UK.

In 2004 the age group with the highest incidence of chlamydia were those under 25 years, and specifically women between 16–19 years and men aged 20–24 years. The risk factors for chlamydia include being young, single, having concurrent sexual partners, having high numbers of sexual partners and unprotected sexual contact (the UK Collaborative Group for HIV and STI Surveillance, 2005).

In what ways would this data assist in sexual health service planning?

The health information in the previous Activity indicates a likely additional demand for sexual health services. It also suggests that services should be targeted at young people with single sex clinics likely to be most effective and acceptable. This increase in chlamydia diagnosis is due in part to an increase in genitourinary medicine (GUM) activity, improved diagnostic techniques, including 'self sampling', greater awareness, and publicity associated with the National Chlamydia

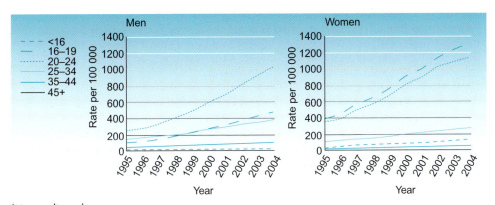

¹Uncomplicated

Figure 7.1   Rates of genital chlamydial¹ infection by sex and age group, UK:1995–2004. The UK Collaborative Group for HIV and STI Surveillance. *Mapping the Issues. HIV and other Sexually Transmitted Infections in the United Kingdom: 2005.* London: Health Protection Agency Centre for Infections. November 2005.

Screening Programme (NCSP). The NCSP focuses on screening asymptomatic men and women under the age of 25 years in a variety of clinical and non-clinical settings where they would not ordinarily be offered chlamydia screening.

Surveillance data can assist in planning an effective health intervention programme encompassing services, education and policy. Table 7.2 is a summary of evidence on effective sexual health programmes which may address service delivery and organisation; information, education and communication; and policy initiatives.

Table 7.2 Effective sexual health programme.

Education	Services	Policy
• Clear 'risk' information • Clear ways to avoid intercourse or protect against STIs and pregnancy • Communication, negotiation and refusal skills practice	• Confidentiality and being non judgemental • Open access, e.g. after school	• Reduce transmission of STIs • Reduce prevalence of undiagnosed HIV and STIs
• Participatory teaching methods and appropriate materials	• Youth friendly staff and environment	• Reduce unintended pregnancy rates
• Active involvement of parents who feel able to discuss relationships and sexual health at home	• Single sex clinics	• Improve the health and social care for people living with HIV
• Help to resist peer pressure to have sex early • Strong leadership	• Awareness of cultural issues • Understanding of the legal framework surrounding those under 16 years	– –
–	• Contraceptive and counselling services that are age appropriate	–
–	• Clear referral pathways to specialist services	–
–	• Free on-site treatment of STIs	–

Source: DoH (2001); Swann *et al* (2003); Tripp and Viner (2005)

Global surveillance

The revised International Health Regulations (IHR) and the World Health Organization (WHO) focus on surveillance and management of conditions of global public health concern. There are two important surveillance networks;

(1) Global Public Health Intelligence Network – computer application that continuously scans the internet for reports of suspicious disease events.

(2) Global Outbreak Alert and Response Network – an operational system for keeping evolving infectious disease threats under close surveillance and facilitating the rapid containment of outbreaks.

Surveillance may be compromised by limited monitoring capacity which may be due to war, natural disaster or poorly funded observational systems. Reporting a disease outbreak may reduce economic viability by impacting on trade, tourism and travel, e.g. in 2003 China delayed reporting the severe acute respiratory syndrome (SARS) outbreak.

Case study 7.1: Influenza surveillance

The potential threat of influenza pandemic from type A/H5N1 currently infecting poultry has highlighted the need for robust surveillance. The concern with A/H5N1 is that it could readily change 'host' and adapt to spread from birds to humans. A new strain also means that populations do not have any immunity and until the virus has been identified no effective vaccine can be manufactured. There are three main groups of influenza – A, B and C – with type A causing all previous pandemics. Types B and C infect humans only but type A has the ability to infect animals and humans. Each year we need a new influenza vaccine to combat the seasonal influenza outbreak as Type A changes its surface antigens in order to produce a different strain of influenza. These minor changes are called 'antigenic drift'. A pandemic can occur when there is a major change in surface antigens resulting in a new influenza strain; this is known as 'antigenic shift'. An influenza pandemic can occur at any time of year, may affect all ages and has far higher rates of morbidity and mortality than ordinary seasonal influenza.

Influenza surveillance is a global, European and national activity which entails monitoring the incidence, distribution and genetic changes of influenza. The agencies involved include the WHO

Continued

Global Influenza Surveillance Network with four collaborating centres in Australia, Japan, USA and UK. The European Influenza Scheme funded by the European Union which monitors influenza data from 23 European countries and the HPA in the UK which monitors circulating influenza strains. The HPA aims to identify new subtypes of influenza with pandemic potential by collecting health information from GPs on 'flu like' illness and laboratory reports which are generated from swabs taken from the nose and throat.

Surveillance, prevention and control of non-communicable diseases

In recognition of the changing pattern of disease, measures are also in place to protect populations from non-communicable disease. Table 7.3 gives some examples of how populations can be protected from non-communicable disease.

The role of the nurse in health protection

A key aspect of the nurse's role in relation to protecting the public is the ability to communicate about risk at an individual and population level. It is necessary to make an assessment of the risk understanding of patients as part of shared decision-making and in order to obtain informed consent. This is because communicating about risk involves

Table 7.3 Protection from non-communicable disease.

Surveillance includes monitoring	Antibiotic resistance to identify emerging strains of antibiotic resistance Prescribing habits of GPs in order to ascertain patterns of prescribing drugs Long-term conditions in diabetics so that they can be detected and managed at an early stage
Health protection policy includes	Fluoridation of water to prevent dental decay The prohibition of smoking in public places in Scotland and Ireland
Clinical practice includes	Folic acid in pregnancy to prevent neural tube defects Septrin to prevent pneumocystis carinii pneumonia (PCP) in HIV positive individuals Statins for those with increased cholesterol levels or other major risk factors for cardiac disease

making choices, e.g., 'should I have this screening test for cancer?' or 'should I have my child vaccinated?' The manner in which the nurse communicates risk affects the patient's perception of risk.

In order to make an assessment of risk the nurse needs to:

(1) elicit beliefs
(2) understand misperceptions
(3) add missing information
(4) correct misinformation
(5) strengthen correct beliefs
(6) de-emphasise unimportant beliefs
(7) praise risk perception
(8) evaluate their communication.

When discussing risk with either groups or individuals the focus of the risk communication needs to be clearly defined. For example when informing about sexual health risk, is the focus:

(1) Lifestyle risk?
(2) Risk of death?
(3) Risk of acquiring HIV with one episode of unprotected sexual intercourse?
(4) Lifetime risk of, e.g. developing ovarian cancer?

Activity

(1) Which is the bigger risk – a 1 in 35 or 1 in 400 chance of developing a disease?
(2) Which choice is more acceptable from the following estimated probabilities? You have 90 out of 100 chance of dying or 10 out of 100 chance of being cured.

Barriers to risk communication occur when there is an ambiguity of risk terms such as 'common' and 'very rare'. Such terms are likely to reflect the speaker's perception rather than being accurate assessments (Paling, 2003). Many people will think that 1 in 400 has a higher probability possibly due to the larger denominator. When giving a probability outcome for different choices you should use the same denominator to lessen confusion. Question 2 is framed to give the same information positively and negatively, however the 10 out of 100 probability will be psychologically more acceptable. When seeking informed consent the nurse should frame probabilities both positively and negatively.

Research (DoH, 1997) has identified that perceptions of risk are biased amongst the public and at times health professionals in the following ways:

- we think our predictions of risk are more accurate than they actually are
- once we have a perception of risk it is difficult to change as we disregard information that does not support our perception
- there is a social amplification of particular events occurring if these have received lots of media coverage
- there is an over estimate of the risk of death due to unusual causes such as floods and an underestimate from those common causes such as CHD.

The impact of the media on shaping risk perception of the public and health professionals alike can be enormous and is frequently misguided. Factors that may distort risk perception include those that are:

- involuntary, e.g. exposure to bird flu is seen as less acceptable than voluntary risks associated with smoking
- from an unfamiliar source
- harmful from an identifiable person (e.g. the Chief Medical Officer) as opposed to an anonymous person
- lacking in scientific understanding
- inescapable from taking personal precautions, e.g. biological warfare.

Perception of risk is also influenced by health information on the internet. To support the nurse in risk communication The National Library for Health (http://www.library.nhs.uk/rss/) is a government health gateway which features a section called 'Hitting the headlines'. This section highlights the most recent media headlines to do with health and should provide up to date, clear and evidence-based information on the subject matter. In order to highlight trustworthy sources of online health and medical information the Health on the Net Foundation (http://www.hon.ch/index.html) provides a code of conduct with eight ethical standards. Credible sources of health information on the net can then display the Health on the Net seal.

The nurse needs to remember that internet sites do not always accurately communicate risk. For example research (Jøgensen and Gøtzsche, 2004) into the presentation on websites from professional advocacy groups (including charities), governmental institutes and consumer groups into the possible benefits and harms from screening for breast cancer found that information on the internet is biased in favour of screening. The advocacy groups and governmental institutions gave an unbalanced representation of the benefits and harms of mammography screening and did not accurately portray over-diagnosis and over-treatment. The public's perception of risk is also shaped by health information from readily available access to health journals such as the

British Medical Journal and the *Nursing Standard*. Access to these sources may impact upon perception in the following ways:

- someone has misinterpreted accurate information
- someone has assimilated inaccurate information
- someone knows as much, if not more, than the nurse.

Summary

This chapter has described key approaches that protect the health of populations, namely vaccination and screening. The monitoring of these programmes and other diseases and conditions has been made visible with reference to the importance of surveillance, both nationally and internationally. Policy and recommended clinical guidance to protect populations from non-communicable disease has also been highlighted. The underpinning principle is that in order to protect the health of populations, individual choice may be eroded and this poses an ethical dilemma for the nurse in practice.

Further reading and resources

The following websites contain information about disease trends and health protection interventions:

Communicable Disease Report (CDR Weekly): http://www.immunisation.org.uk

Department of Health Pandemic flu: http:// www.dh.gov.uk/pandemicflu

Health on the Net foundation: http://www.hon.ch/index.html.

Health Protection Agency: http://www.hpa.org.uk

London Health Observatory: http://www.lho.org.uk

National Electronic Library for Screening – National Screening Committees policy position on screening for individual conditions: http://www.nelh.nhs.uk/screening

National Library for Health: http://www.library.nhs.uk/rss/.

NHS Screening – website containing screening information for health professionals in the UK: www.screening.nhs.uk

UK National Screening Committees: http://www.nsc.nhs.uk

World Health Organization UK Immunization profile: http://www.who.int/immunization-monitoring.

References

Cribb A. and Duncan P. (2002) *Health Promotion and Professional Ethics*. Oxford, Blackwell Publishing Ltd.

Department of Health (1997) *Communicating about risks to public health: Pointers to good practice*. DoH, London.

Department of Health (2001) *Better prevention better services better sexual health. The National Sexual Health and HIV strategy*. DoH, London.

Department of Health (2002) *Getting Ahead of the Curve*. HMSO, London.

Department of Health (2003) *Evaluation of English Bowel (Colorectal) Cancer Screening Pilot*. Accessed online http://www.cancerscreening.nhs.uk/bowel/pilot-evaluation.html.

Department of Health (2005) *Vaccination services reducing inequalities in uptake*. DoH, London.

Health Protection Agency (2004) *Supplementary data tables of the Unlinked Anonymous Prevalence Monitoring Programme: data to the end of 2003. Surveillance Update 2004*. HPA, London.

Jøgensen K. and Gøtzsche P. (2004) Presentation on websites of possible benefits and harms from screening for breast cancer: cross sectional study, *British Medical Journal*, **328**, 148–52.

Kirk M. (2005) Tailoring genetic information and services to clients' culture, knowledge and language level, *Nursing Standard*, **20**, 2, 52–6.

Lewendon G. and Maconachie M. (2002) Why are children not being immunised? Barriers to immunisation uptake in South Devon, *Health Education Journal*, **61**, 3, 212–220.

National Institute for Clinical Excellence (2004) *Depression: Management of Depression in Primary and Secondary Care*. NICE, London.

Paling J. (2003) Strategies to help patients understand risks, *British Medical Journal*, **327**, 745–87.

Summerfield D. (2006) Depression: epidemic or pseudo-epidemic? *Journal of The Royal Society of Medicine*, **99**, 1–2.

Swann C. Bowe K. Mc Cormick G. and Kosmin M. (2003) *Teenage pregnancy and parenthood: a review of reviews. Evidence briefing* London, Health Development Agency.

The UK Collaborative Group for HIV and STI Surveillance (2005) *Mapping the Issues. HIV and other Sexually Transmitted Infections in the United Kingdom: 2005*. Health Protection Agency Centre for Infections, London.

Tripp J. and Viner R. (2005) Sexual health, contraception, and teenage pregnancy, *British Medical Journal*, **330**, 590–3.

UK National Screening Committee (2000) *Second Report*. DoH, London.

UK Public Health Association (2005) *Choosing or Losing Health?* UKPHA, London.

Promoting Healthy Lifestyles

Jenny Husbands

Introduction

Previous chapters have shown how health and disease are determined by many factors that interact together, yet health behaviours and lifestyles are responsible for a considerable burden of ill-health and disease. Because treatment has become expensive and often of questionable efficacy in health improvement and because genetic factors are largely unalterable, the focus has shifted to encouraging changes to individual lifestyles. This chapter is concerned with what people believe and how they behave in relation to their health. The chapter explores the ways in which nurses may help individuals to change their behaviour through advice and information, counselling and through education.

Learning outcomes

By the end of this chapter you will be able to:

- identify how lifestyles influence health behaviour and health status
- understand how people make choices about their health
- discuss the role of the nurse in encouraging and supporting people to change.

Healthy lifestyles

The threat of childhood death from illness is falling and the big infectious killer diseases of the last century have been eradicated or largely controlled, but deaths from cancers, coronary heart disease (CHD) and stroke have risen. They now account for around two-thirds of all deaths. Cancer, stroke and heart disease not only kill, but are also major causes of ill-health, preventing people from living their lives to the full and causing avoidable disability, pain and anxiety. These diseases are largely preventable as their greatest risk factors arise from individual behaviours and the way that people lead their lives.

- Smoking remains the single biggest preventable cause of ill-health and there are approximately 114 000 premature deaths from smoking in the UK every day. Most deaths from smoking are related to lung cancer, CHD and chronic obstructive pulmonary disease (Doll *et al*, 1994; Peto *et al*, 2003).
- As many as one in ten sexually active young women may be infected with chlamydia, which can cause infertility. Chlamydia rates have risen steadily, with over 82 000 diagnoses being made in 2002 (HPA, 2003).
- 1 in every 250 pregnant women in London is HIV positive (HPA, 2003).
- Alcohol is a factor in 20–30% of accidents and thus places a particular strain on accident and emergency departments. Alcohol related deaths cause between 20 000–40 000 deaths in England and Wales from stroke, cancer and liver disease annually (DoH, 2001).
- Obesity has nearly trebled in the UK since the 1980s. It is associated with increased risk of CHD, cancer, diabetes and stroke and high blood pressure. An estimated 50% of the adult population are over weight and 20% of the adult population are obese (House of Commons Select Committee, 2004).
- Levels of physical activity remain at dangerously low levels, indeed it is estimated that 70% of the adult population do not participate in sufficient physical activity levels to contribute to health gain and this is associated with diseases such as coronary vascular disease, diabetes mellitus, hypertension and strokes and skeletal disorders such as osteoporosis and osteoarthritis (DoH, 2004).

The traditional focus of health promotion has been on modifying those behaviours such as smoking and diet that are known to have an impact on people's health. The English national public health strategy 'Our Healthier Nation' (DoH, 1998) identified aspects of individual behaviour as risk factors for particular conditions and set targets to reduce those behaviours by 2010. These targets are:

- to reduce deaths from heart disease and strokes amongst people under 65 years by one-third
- to reduce deaths from accidents by one-fifth
- to reduce mental ill-health and deaths from suicide by one-sixth
- to reduce deaths from cancer by one-fifth.

Activity

Identify the known risk factors for CHD.
Which of these are linked to individual behaviours?

The risk factors for CHD are smoking, inactivity, eating a diet high in saturated fat, excessive alcohol consumption, type 2 diabetes, hypertension, genetics/family history, socio-economic status, gender and age. Some of these factors are known as intrinsic factors, e.g. age, gender and family history/genetics and these factors are not associated with individual behaviour. However, some factors known as extrinsic factors such as smoking, drinking excessive amounts of alcohol, eating a high saturated fat diet and physical inactivity are classed as health damaging behaviour that the individual has some control over.

There are many influences on people's behaviour. Whether people take part in physical activity, for example, may be influenced by:

- gender (fewer women than men exercise)
- age (activity levels decline with age)
- beliefs such as 'not being the sporty type'
- concern about body image
- lack of time
- culture (some cultures view physical activity as a low priority or unacceptable)
- socio-economic class (some of the lower socio-economic groups may be unable to participate in physical activity due to financial barriers).

Even when we know what would be healthy choices, we don't necessarily choose them. All sorts of factors influence the choices we make. People respond to the social context in which they live and may participate in health damaging behaviours in order to cope with the pressures of their everyday lives. Graham (1993), for example, found in her studies about women and smoking, that women from lower socio-economic groups reported that it was the only thing they had for themselves in a world of insurmountable difficulties. Marsh and McKay (1994) found that 70% of lone parents smoke compared to 28% of the rest of the population. Many nurses feel that smoking is their only pleasure in an otherwise stressful day and allows them to acquire their much needed breaks (McKenna *et al*, 2003).

Protective health behaviours are also less common amongst people living in disadvantaged circumstances. It is not simply that people do not know that their health behaviour is damaging to their health, but access to and availability of healthy opportunities such as exercise facilities or fresh fruit and vegetables may be less obtainable. The Whitehall Study of civil servants found that lower grades report more stress and have less social support and personal resources to deal with the sources of stress (Cabinet Office, 1997).

Health decision making

Part of the nurse's health promotion role is to encourage people to adopt healthier lifestyles. To do this it is important to think through what influences whether or not people make changes to their health and health behaviour. A key element in people's behaviour is their attitude to that behaviour. People's attitudes are made up of two components:

- cognitive – the knowledge and information which contribute to their beliefs about the behaviour
- affective – their emotions and values about what is of importance.

Activity

Think of a health behaviour that you may want to change.
What knowledge or information may influence you?
How does your attitude to the behaviour influence what you do?

A person's attitudes will also be influenced by:

- their past experiences of and attitudes towards health and social care provision
- their previous successes or failures to change their behaviour and lifestyle
- the support they received from both their family and friends and health and social care providers
- their perceptions of, or health beliefs about their illness or disease
- their gender, age, culture and socio-economic group.

A person's skills will also influence their ability and desire to change their health behaviour and lifestyle. If, for example, the individual wants to change their level of physical activity and starts off by par-

Individual perceptions   Modifying factors   Likelihood of action

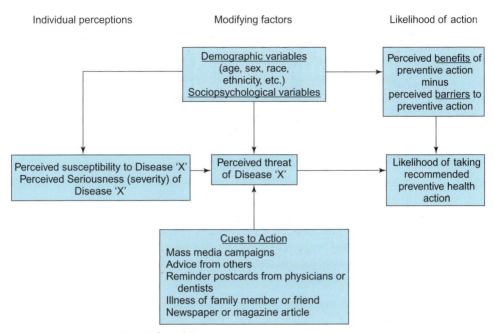

Figure 8.1 The Health Belief Model.

ticipating in a high impact, vigorous activity which requires a high level of skill, after previously leading a sedentary lifestyle, their lack of skill may result in injury and therefore prevent them from any future involvement in that or any other activity.

A patient's knowledge will also influence their ability to change their behaviour and lifestyle. For example, a patient may wish to change their eating patterns and adopt a healthier way of eating. However, they may be unsure of the healthy eating messages in terms of frequency, amount and types of healthy foods and therefore may feel too overwhelmed to change their current eating patterns.

One way of understanding how people make decisions about their health behaviour and lifestyle is to use a model of health behaviour. Figure 8.1, Becker's Health Belief Model (1974), illustrates the elements involved in individual decision making about health and whether the individual believes themselves to be:

- susceptible or at risk
- at a severe health risk because the consequences of not taking action would be severe
- capable of taking action.

Perceived susceptibility

This is based on the subjective perception of the risk of developing a condition, illness or disease; i.e. does the individual believe that they are at real risk of developing an illness? Most people think they are less likely to get a problem than other people and nurses may hear patients say things like 'People like me don't get that.'

Perceived severity

This relates to feelings about the seriousness of contracting an illness or leaving an illness untreated; i.e. is leaving the illness untreated worse than the illness itself? People will not consider the consequences as serious if they believe it can be prevented by taking action at some point in the future or if any outcomes are likely to be some time ahead. Nurses may hear patients say 'You've got to die sometime' or 'I'll worry when the time comes'.

Perceived benefits

An individual must believe that an action will be effective in reducing the severity of the illness and that there are definite benefits in taking that action; i.e. having a child immunised. Nurses may hear patients say 'I would rather stop my child getting one of those awful diseases'.

Perceived barriers

An individual may cite a lack of time, lack of access, costs or negative perceptions associated with the behaviour that will deter them from embarking on a health behaviour change. Nurses may hear patients say 'If I give up smoking I'll put on weight' or 'I won't be able to cope with stress if I stop smoking.'

A person may also need some sort of push or incentive to start thinking about making a change. This might be:

- a change in circumstances, e.g. a pregnancy might prompt a reduction in drinking
- new information, e.g. a doctor performing a liver function test might prompt a reduction in drinking
- the passage of time, e.g. older people feeling less mobile might be prompted to be more active
- a significant other may develop an illness related to their health behaviour which may trigger a patient to take stock of their own health behaviour.

Activity

Think back to a time in your life when you wanted to change your health behaviour/lifestyle, e.g. giving up smoking, increasing your levels of physical activity, eating more healthily, decreasing your alcohol consumption. Did you:

(1)   Consider your risk of developing an illness or disease?
(2)   Consider the seriousness of the illness or disease?
(3)   Weigh up the pros and cons of making a change, e.g. what were the benefits? What were the costs?
(4)   Did you succeed in making the change? What helped you?

Some people find it easier to make a change than others. The concept of a health locus of control distinguishes between those with an:

- internal locus of control – people who see their health as largely within their own control. These people are more likely to adopt activities to enhance their health
- external locus of control – people who see their health as a matter of chance and so outside their control. These people are more likely to adopt health damaging behaviours than those with an internal locus of control.

The following scenario illustrates some of the factors influencing patients' confidence and ability to change their lifestyle and health behaviour.

Scenario

Margo is 40 years and has been dieting and exercising infrequently for the past 20 years. Recently Margo's weight has begun to creep up and she finds it increasingly difficult to walk up the stairs.

Margo decides to try the latest diet fad that she saw on breakfast television and goes back to the gym to do spinning classes. The first three days of her new diet go well and although she feels hungry she feels able to cope with this as she notices that she has lost 2lbs.

When Margo goes to the spinning class she finds it very difficult, she is unable to keep up with the rest of the group and she feels weak and dizzy afterwards. Feeling a little deflated Margo goes home and eats a bar of chocolate to give herself energy (she tells herself that it doesn't matter as she has lost 2lbs anyway).

Continued

> Margo feels unable to face another gruelling spinning class and decides to give the gym a miss, she feels unsupported by her family and friends who neither offer support or encouragement with her efforts to lose weight.
>
> The practice nurse at her general practitioner (GP) surgery meets Margo when she attends for a smear test and they discuss general health concerns.
>
> What could the nurse do to support Margo in her attempts to lose weight?

People are motivated to take action when they feel the outcome is likely to be valuable or beneficial and when they feel they can do it effectively. Several factors affect people's feelings of self efficacy and whether they think they can change:

- perceptions of their own will power
- whether they have enough relevant information
- perceptions of their own coping skills
- whether they feel supported by family and friends.

Cavill *et al* (2006) found that brief advice from a health professional which is supported by written material such as health education leaflets can be effective in producing modest short-term (6–12 weeks) effect on physical activity. If the patient was referred to a community-based exercise specialist the results could last eight months.

Approaches to changing lifestyles

Health promotion is everybody's business and can have a positive impact on the work of the nurse and their patient's health. For example, during a routine contact with a patient the nurse can use this time to discuss:

- any concerns the patient may have with their health
- what needs the patient has
- what other influences there are on the patient's health
- what behaviour changes they may wish to make.

The nurse can use this time to give brief health promotion interventions. This may result not only in the patient feeling valued and listened to, but also give the patient a feeling of control over their own health. If patients feel more in control of their life, they are more likely to feel enabled to make health choices and feel empowered to take part in their own care planning. A range of activities can be used by the nurse to promote health. Such examples include:

- one-to-one discussions – these can be carried out by the nurse at the patient's bedside; during out-patient's appointments; during primary care appointments; in the patient's home. For example, the student nurse gives advice on healthy eating to a patient whilst discharging the patient from hospital who had been admitted with unstable diabetes mellitus
- group discussions – these can be carried out by the nurse during in-patient stays in hospital; during health promotion groups such as antenatal classes; or during primary care clinics. For example, the student nurse helps to facilitate an antenatal class with the community nurse as part of her maternity placement and gives advice on healthy eating in pregnancy
- telephone contacts – these can be carried out by the nurse from the ward or community setting as a means of making contact or keeping in contact with patients. For example, the student nurse on community placement follows up patients who have attended the health promotion group on healthy eating to offer support and encouragement
- disseminating information and explanation leaflets – this can be carried out by the nurse during in-patient episodes; whilst discharging patients; during health promotion groups and health fairs; and in the community. For example, the student nurse gives patients health education leaflets and gives health education advice as part of their discharge information in order to encourage patients to change their health behaviour
- health stalls – these can be carried out by the student nurse as part of community placement. For example, a student nurse sets up a health stall in the hospital foyer to provide information on smoking cessation groups as part of National No Smoking Day

In order to be able to carry out health promotion interventions key skills are required in:

- information giving
- communication
- counselling
- education.

Information giving

Explaining is a core skill that is often challenging for the nurse and poor information giving is a common source of patient dissatisfaction. As well as giving information about treatments and procedures, the nurse may need to give information about behaviour changes such as healthy eating or reducing alcohol consumption. The nurse has to be able to give information in a manner that is acceptable, understandable, coherent, safe and appropriate. The nurse should also be giving advice that is contemporaneous and evidence-based. The key features of effective information giving are:

- tailoring information to what a patient needs to know
- checking the patient's understanding
- eliciting reactions to the information.

Written information may be used to reinforce verbal information. The presentation of health information should be appropriate, understandable, accurate, acceptable (as much as possible), visually appealing, clear and precise. Again this should be based on contemporaneous and evidence-based information. Figure 8.2 shows a page from a leaflet on sensible drinking produced by the Health Education Board for Scotland (2003). All leaflets should be appraised for their suitability before using them with patients.

Ewles and Simnett (2003) devised a checklist to help nurses and other health promoters to appraise health promotion leaflets:

- Is the leaflet brief and to the point?
- Does the leaflet emphasise the key points?
- Does the leaflet use language that is easy to understand?
- Are the words and images easy to see?
- Is the design of the leaflet visually appealing, e.g. colour, images and size?
- How could you use the leaflet to make an effective display?

Activity

Using the checklist devised by Ewles and Simnett (2003) appraise a leaflet (these are easily available in primary care centres or online at http://hebs.scot.nhs.uk or http://doh.gov.uk).

Think about how you could use it to promote health with your patients.

Patient information services, which aim to enable patients to make informed choices have expanded recently and include services such as:

- NHS Direct which is a 24 hour nurse-led telephone advisory service
- Centre for Health Information Quality which is a resource for disseminating and producing high quality patient information and focuses on providing information on treatment choices and outcomes
- organising Medical Networked Information which is an organisation that provides access to good quality biomedical and health information from the internet

drinking and driving

Recent statistics show that about 15,000 people are injured and 500 are killed in the UK every year as a result of drinking and driving. One in three of the drivers killed in road traffic accidents have blood alcohol levels over the legal limit.

What is the legal limit?

The law says that it is an offence to drive with more than 80mg of alcohol in every 100ml of blood. It's best just not to drink at all if you are going to drive.

But how does drink affect you?

There is no simple answer to this question. How alcohol affects you depends a lot on your age, gender, whether or not you have eaten anything and if you are taking other drugs. It's best just not to drink at all if you are going to drive.

Can you tell if you are safe to drive?

You can't. Alcohol affects your mind. It makes you feel more confident, so you are less likely to make a balanced decision about whether or not to drive.

It also reduces your inhibitions so you may be more likely to take risks and to react violently when you are driving.

How does alcohol affect driving?

Alcohol slows down the brain and so:

- your ability to concentrate will be reduced

- your ability to judge speed and distance, and to deal with the unexpected, will be impaired

- your reaction time will be lengthened

- your vision and awareness will become blurred, especially in the dark

- your can lose muscle control and coordination.

All this means that you are far more likely to have an accident.

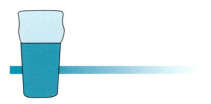

Figure 8.2   Alcohol facts – a guide to sensible drinking, available at http://www.hebs.scot.nhs.uk/services/pubs/pdf/Alcofacts.pdf. © produced with kind permission of NHS Health Scotland.

- Patient UK which was designed for non-medical people and provides information about health related issues (Coulter *et al*, 1999; Sheppard *et al*, 1999).

Communication

Good communication in health promotion is important because it enables the nurse to successfully deliver clear, concise unmistakable health promotion messages.

Health promotion communication can take place in any setting and at any time, for example:

- on the ward during admission or discharge of the patient
- before a procedure such as changing a dressing
- during visiting time when the nurse discusses the patient's care with their relatives
- as part of the rehabilitation process for patients with long-term conditions such as diabetes mellitus.

Communication can be difficult at times for a number of reasons such as:

- when the first language of patient and nurse differ
- when the patient is hard of hearing or deaf
- when the patient has a number of presenting problems and may be unable to take on new information
- when the nurses are busy and therefore do not convey messages effectively
- when nurses use jargon
- when the health information is unrealistic or appears to be irrelevant.

In order to communicate effectively with patients and engage in active listening nurses must use a range of communication skills known collectively as **SOLER** which means:

- **S**it squarely facing the patient, ideally on the same level
- **O**pen questions
- **L**isten actively to the patient
- **E**ye contact if acceptable to the patient
- **R**eflection, i.e. repeat the wishes expressed by the patient back to them to clarify that the nurse has heard and understood the patient's expressed needs.

The nurse needs to demonstrate respect for the individual and maintenance of the patient's dignity at all times.

> **Activity**
>
> Ines has been admitted to your ward with an acute asthmatic attack. Ines lives in temporary accommodation and has no relatives in London. She speaks little English and appears frightened and confused.
>
> What could the nurse do to allay some of Ines' fears?
> What would be the most helpful strategies for the nurse to use in order to assess Ines' needs?
> What would be unhelpful communication strategies?

As a nurse, it is important to take into account the cultural and social needs of your patients and take on board the impact this may have on their ability to accept and/or interpret the health information you give them. Some possible solutions that may address Ines' fears include providing information in a format that she is able to understand and that she finds acceptable. This health information should include advice that takes into account her social and psychological health as well as her physical health needs.

Some useful strategies that the nurse could employ include utilising interpreting and advocacy services; the former will translate information from the nurse to the patient and vice versa; the latter will act on Ines' behalf to ensure that doctors and nurses and other health and social care providers meet Ines' needs and enable her to make informed health choices. Nurses should ensure that their communication with patients whose first language is not English is not unhelpful and disempowering, e.g.

* speaking very loudly in order to be understood
* using inappropriate interpreters such as ancillary staff from similar ethnic backgrounds
* making health decisions on behalf of their patients without involving the patient in the process
* disseminating written health promotion literature in a language that the patient is unable to understand
* failing to make any attempt to communicate with their patient because they do not speak the same language (Lea, 1994; Dosani, 2001).

Counselling

Counselling approaches aim to work with the patient in relation to their own health agenda. They place the patient at the centre of the intervention and the nurse takes on the role of facilitator and empowerer. For example, the nurse will enable the patient to decide on their own course of health action and support them in this, rather than setting the health agenda. A patient who does not express a wish to

realistic objectives/actions and is time specific, i.e. will start on a specific date or to be for a specific time span.

- **Maintaining change** is the next stage and is when most people are working to prevent a relapse or recurrence of their old health behaviour. This may be because of the external pressures on the person. This stage is said to be one of the hardest for the patient and they are said to have succeeded if they can maintain the behaviour for a lengthy period of time depending on the behaviour. For example, not smoking for six months, being physically active for eight weeks. In other words the new health behaviour has become habitual. The strategy employed here by the nurse would be to encourage the patient to reward themselves for being able to maintain the new health behaviour (obviously not with a reward that would sabotage their efforts).
- **Relapse** may be the next stage and is said to occur when the patient is unable to sustain the new health behaviour for numerous reasons, such as: bereavement; stress; changed circumstances; lack of support; boredom; lack of incentives; lack of motivation, etc. Relapse is a normal component of behaviour change and Prochaska and DiClemente (1992) argue that the patient should not think of themselves as a failure. The nurse's strategy here would be to use this opportunity to review with the patient their action plan to see if it was realistic or too over ambitious. It is important to help the patient to understand that relapse is not failure, but a normal part of the process of change.

Figure 8.3 shows how these theoretical models on individual behaviour change have been applied to guidance on smoking cessation and recommendations for brief interventions in primary care.

Such client centred approaches arguably need specific characteristics on the part of the nurse which Carl Rogers (1951) called core qualities. These core qualities help patients in a therapeutic relationship with the nurse and include:

- Unconditional positive regard – acceptance of people irrespective of their condition, age, gender, culture, ethnicity, socio-economic background, expressed thoughts, behaviours or beliefs. The patient should not be judged by any set of rules or standards. The nurse must set aside their own values and beliefs, biases and prejudices in order to help their patient. This acceptance should not be confused with liking or approval of the patient.
- Genuineness or congruence – this means being oneself or being true and sincere, being non-defensive and free in behaviour and being real. The nurse would therefore use their own language and own behaviour and be genuine.

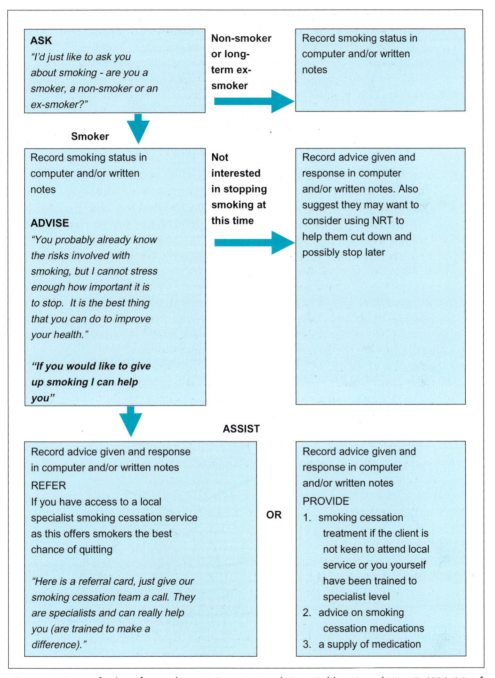

Figure 8.3 Brief advice for smokers. McEwen A. Hajek P. McRobbie H. and West R. (2006) Brief interventions. In McEwen A. Hajek P. McRobbie H. and West R. Manual of Smoking Cessation. A guide for councellors and practitioners. Oxford, Blackwell Publishing Ltd.

- Empathy – this means being able to appreciate the patient's own meanings and understand the world as seen through the eyes of the patient.

Thus the focus of the intervention is to take on board the patient's 'frame of reference' and to endeavour to understand the patient and appreciate their circumstance from their perspective; to enable and encourage the patient to take responsibility for their own health decisions and actions. Rogers (1951) argues that if the above is in place then behaviour change is more likely to happen.

Activity

A patient on your ward is about to be discharged after an admission for chronic bronchitis. He is aged 60 years and has smoked 40 cigarettes a day for over 40 years. He is worried about his health and has expressed an interest in changing his health behaviour.

Using the Stages of Change model (Prochaska and DiClemente, 1992) what questions would you ask to assess their readiness to change?
What strategies could you employ to support your patient?
What influences on his health would you need to consider?
What core qualities would you need to use to facilitate behaviour change by the patient?

The nurse could ask the patient to consider the benefits and the cost factor related to their current health behaviour; if the benefits outweigh the cost, then it's safe to assume they are ready to change. The nurse should give patients the opportunity to discuss their smoking habit and if the nurse does not feel confident to support the patient, refer them (with their consent) to a smoking cessation specialist. The nurse should also encourage patients to discuss any concerns they may have about becoming a non-smoker and the support networks they may have around them. The nurse and the patient should also consider the risk the patient faces from their current health behaviour, such as hypertension. In terms of evidence of effectiveness, it is important to consider that patients may relapse several times before they become a non-smoker but that support from a GP or nurse is valuable for a successful outcome (Fiore *et al*, 2000). In addition, nurses need to consider the reasons why patients smoke and take into account their socio-economic situation.

Education

Educational approaches to health promotion are important because they aim not merely to give people information but to give people an informed choice and to help them to acquire knowledge and skills in order to make that choice. With this approach, education or information is presented and patients are encouraged to explore their own attitudes, skills and knowledge about their health. Patients may also be assisted to help make changes to their lifestyle. For example, a nurse will give patients information on healthy eating; may help the patient to explore their attitudes and knowledge about what constitutes a healthy diet and may escort the patient to a local supermarket to identify healthy food choices.

Educational approaches to health promotion take place in a number of settings, for example:

- health promotion clinics in hospital out-patients departments or GP surgeries
- on wards when nurses demonstrate to patients how to look after their stomas
- on wards during admission when a patient is shown how to participate in their care
- on wards during the patient's discharge from hospital when the patient is shown how to self medicate correctly and safely
- in the community, e.g. in the patient's home, GP surgeries or community centres.

For an educational approach to be effective it has to:

- involve using reinforcement
- give feedback
- offer the opportunity for individualisation
- facilitate behaviour change through the use of skills and resources
- ensure that the education/topic must be relevant to the needs of the patient (Mullen, 1992).

Case study 8.1: Effective education in prisons and offending institutions

In the UK considerable attention has been paid to communicable diseases amongst prisoners particularly blood borne viruses, hepatitis C, B and A, and human immunodeficiency virus (HIV). These may be acquired sexually or through substance misuse. Educational models including the following have been shown to be successful.

A programme with recently released parolees from a US prison was based on a social learning approach and included the use of role models and social support as well as job training and out reach work to increase resistance to intravenous (IV) drug taking and drug related behaviours. The results were that a year after being on the programme, parolees demonstrated that they were more

Continued

adjusted to the community and demonstrated fewer drug related behaviours (Wexler *et al*, 1994).

An acquired immune deficiency syndrome (AIDS) prevention training programme for parolees recently released from prison with histories of drug injection was developed and evaluated. Key programme elements included: a social learning approach to prevention which emphasised resistance skills training; a self help orientation stressing individual responsibility; therapeutic community principles such as credible role models and community building; and job readiness training for the AIDS prevention/outreach field. A total of 394 eligible parolees (81% male, 19% female) were recruited, of whom 241 attended the programme including 164 completers. One year follow-up results showed that ARRIVE (the programme title) participation significantly decreased certain sexual and drug related risk behaviours and improved parolees' community adjustment (Williamson, 2006).

Scenario:

A young mothers group

Group members of a young mothers group wanted to know about a safe, effective and inexpensive physical activity to help them to lose weight. The coordinator and the group members drew up a programme which included the following learning outcomes, learning methods and evaluation of objectives.

Learning outcomes:

- know what types of activity are safe and effective
- explore attitudes and beliefs about different activities
- know physical activity opportunities available locally
- consider the gaps in knowledge and skills about physical activity in order to promote activity with their families.

Learning methods:

- keep activity diaries
- group discussion of experiences, attitudes and beliefs
- group to disseminate information of opportunities, access and availability of physical activity options.

Evaluation of objectives:

- group would be able to describe safe and effective methods of physical activity
- group would be aware of a range of available options locally
- group would be participating in physical activity
- group would feel confident about promoting physical activity with their families.

This scenario illustrates how an educational approach to health promotion can be used in a community setting with patients and that this approach can be acceptable to patients and empower patients by giving them health choices. This may have the added value of giving patients more confidence in their ability to make behaviour and lifestyle changes, but it must be noted that this has to be considered in the context in which patients live and their ability to make health choices.

The role of the nurse in promoting health behaviour and lifestyle change

Changing health behaviour and lifestyles can be a very daunting challenge for the nurse who has to integrate health promotion into their other work. The student nurse has to learn many technical procedures, skills and theoretical concepts and may find health promotion too difficult a concept to apply to their everyday tasks. Although initially the nurse may not see relevance or importance of health promotion in their work, aiming to change health behaviour can have a much wider impact than on the health of the individual patient. For example if patients feel enabled and empowered, they may try to influence the health of their families, friends and communities. This knock-on effect could arguably be seen as primary prevention, i.e. addressing the health needs of the population before the onset of disease or illness.

Encouraging people to change their health behaviour and lifestyle can be viewed by the patient and public at large as interfering and controlling. Victim blaming is unhelpful and nurses could make some people feel that they are being blamed for their ill-health and health damaging lifestyle and that it is their sole responsibility to adapt health enhancing behaviour. Blaming the victim may encourage people to give up the one coping mechanism they have in their lives, but it may not significantly improve their health; or it may exacerbate the patient's socio-economic situation, by making the patient feel responsible for their ill-health and may result in the patient failing to take on board health messages as they may feel unable to change their health behaviour.

Nurses need to be aware of the impact and influence they have on their patients and be careful about how they convey health messages that encourage changes to health behaviour. Additionally, nurses need to be aware of the other influences on health that are beyond the reach or control of their patients and aim to address those influences using all the power and influence at their disposal.

So what is the nurse's role in changing health behaviour?

- Understanding the principles of health beliefs and how they impact on patients' health behaviour; this includes having an understanding of how patients make health behaviour decisions and the influences on their health.
- Giving health information and advice; this advice should be safe, effective, appropriate and acceptable to the patients.
- Using health information and resources appropriately and in a measured way, for example not just giving out leaflets and flyers to patients but ensuring that you explain the content and enable patients to ask questions.
- Ensuring that health information is contemporaneous and evidence-based. It is your professional responsibility to ensure that all advice and information you give is up to date and evidence-based.
- Empowering patients through education to enable patients to make health choices; by giving patients the full picture and ensuring that they are aware of their options the nurse can feel confident that patients are empowered to make an informed health decision.
- Helping patients to acquire knowledge and skills about the things that affect their health.
- Practically assisting patients to enable them to make health choices; this could be acting as an advocate when patients are given health information and feel unable to express their needs or representing patients' needs to health and social service organisations.
- Using core qualities such as unconditional positive regard, genuineness and empathy; this means nurses using their counselling skills to make patients feel valued, cared for and understood.
- Identifying patients who are ready to change their health behaviour; this would entail nurses targeting those patients and employing strategies that would enable the patient to change their health behaviour.
- Understanding the wider social context in which their patients live and the influence this has on their ability to make health and lifestyle choices; this would include an understanding of people's socio-economic status, housing, employment, etc. and the impact of these on their ability to change their health behaviour.

Summary

This chapter discussed the influences on lifestyle and health behaviour. Promoting healthy behaviours is a core component of the nurse's role and demands particular skills in information giving, communication, counselling and education. What is evident is that there is no one approach to health behaviour change that could be used in all situations and with all patients to meet their individual needs. The health promotion approach used by nurses must be appropriate, evidence-based, acceptable and patient-centred. Nurses have to develop skills and knowledge in order to use health promotion appropriately to aid health behaviour change.

Further reading and resources

Department of Health (2004) *Choosing Health: Making Health Choices Easier.* DoH, London.

This White Paper on public health identifies the ways in which health professionals should work with individuals and some new strategies for motivation in communities such as health trainers.

Ewles L. and Simnett I. (2003) *Promoting Health. A Practical Guide* 5th ed. London, Ballière Tindall.

This long established text provides clear guides for practitioners on how to work with individuals and groups.

Naidoo J. and Wills J. (2000) *Health Promotion: Foundations for Practice* 2nd ed. London, Ballière Tindall.

An easy to read textbook that provides the theoretical basis and principles underpinning health promotion work.

Rollnick S. Mason P. and Butler C. (1999) *Health Behavior Change: A Guide for Practitioners.* London, Churchill Livingstone.

A readable guide on motivational interviewing techniques with lots of case studies and practical guidance.

Department of Health: http://www.doh.gov.uk.

Health Education Board for Scotland: http://hebs.scot.nhs.uk.

References

Becker MH. (1974) *The Health Belief Model and Personal Health Behaviour.* New Jersey, Slack Thorofare.

Cabinet Office (1997) *Work Stress and Health: The Whitehall II Study.* London Public and Commercial Services Union, London.

Cavill N. Buxton K. Bull F. and Foster C. (2006) *Promotion of Physical Activity Among Adults: Evidence into Practice Briefing.* London, NIHCE.

Coulter A. Entwistle V. and Gilbert D. (1999) Sharing Decisions with Patients: Is the Information Good Enough? *British Medical Journal,* **318**, 318–22.

Department of Health (1998) *Saving Lives: Our Healthier Nation.* DoH, London.

Department of Health (2001) *Annual Report of the Chief Medical Officer of the Department of Health.* DoH, London.

Department of Health (2004) *Choosing Health: Making Healthy Choices Easier.* DoH, London.

Dosani S. (2001) How to Practise Medicine in a Multicultural Society *Student British Medical Journal,* **9**, 357–98.

Doll R. Peto R. and Wheatley K. (1994) Mortality in Relation to Smoking: 40 Years' Observation in Male British Doctors, *British Medical Journal,* **309**, 901–11.

Ewles L. and Simnett I. (2003) *Promoting Health. A Practical Guide* 5th ed (p 208–9). London, Ballière Tindall.

Fiore MC. Bailey WC. and Cohen SJ. (2000) *Treating Tobacco Use and Dependence: Clinical Practice Guideline,* Rockville, US Dept of Health and Human Services Public Health Service. In Kerr J. Weitkunat R. and Moretti M. (2005) *ABC of Behaviour Change: A Guide to Successful Disease Prevention and Health Promotion.* London, Elsevier.

Graham H. (1993) *Hardship and Health in Women's Lives.* London, Wheatsheaf.

Health Education Board for Scotland (2003) *Alcofacts. A guide to sensible drinking.* Accessed online http://www.hebs.scot.nhs.uk/services/pubs/pdf/Alcofacts.pdf.

Health Protection Agency (2003) *Annual Report: HIV/AIDS and Other Sexually Transmitted Infections in the UK in 2002.* HPA, London.

House of Commons Select Committee (2004) *Obesity.* The Stationery Office, London.

Lea A. (1994) Nursing in Today's Multicultural Society: A Transcultural Perspective, *Journal of Advanced Nursing,* **20**, 307–13.

Marsh A. and McKay S. (1994) *Poor Smokers.* London Policy Studies Institute, London.

McEwen A. Hajek P. McRobbie H. and West R. (2006) Brief interventions. In McEwen A. Hajek P. McRobbie H. and West R. Manual of Smoking Cessation. A guide for councellors and practitioners. Oxford, Blackwell Publishing Ltd.

McKenna H. Slater P. McCance T. Bunting B. Spiers A. and McElwee G. (2003) The Role of Stress, Peer Influence and Education Levels on the Smoking Behaviour of Nurses, *International Journal of Nursing Studies*, **40**, 359–66.

Mullen PD. Maind DA. and Velez R. (1992) A Meta-Analysis of Controlled Trials of Cardiac Patient Education, *Patient Education and Counselling*, **19**, 143–62.

Peto R. Lopez A. and Boreham J. (2003) *Mortality from Smoking in Developed Countries 1950–2000* 2nd ed. Oxford, OUP.

Prochaska JO. DiClemente CC. and Worcross JC. (1992) In Search of How People Change: Applications to the Addictive Behaviours, *American Psychologist*, **47**, 9, 1102–14.

Rogers C. (1951) *Client Centred Therapy.* Boston, Houghton Mifflin.

Sheppard S. Charnock D. and Gann B. (1999) Helping Patients Access High Quality Health Information, *British Medical Journal*, **319**, 764–6.

Wexler HK. Magura S. Beardsley MM. and Josepher H. (1994) ARRIVE: An AIDS Education/Relapse Prevention Model for High Risk Parolees, *International Journal of Addiction*, **29**, 3, 361–86 cited by Williamson M. (2006) *Improving the Health and Social Outcomes of People Recently Released from Prisons in the UK – A Perspective from Primary Care.* London, Sainsbury Centre for Mental Health.

Williamson M. (2006) *Improving the Health and Social Outcomes of People Recently Released from Prisons in the UK – A Perspective from Primary Care.* London, Sainsbury Centre for Mental Health.

Promoting Health for Communities

Linda Jackson

Introduction

The number of registered nurses employed by Primary Care Trusts (PCTs) and general practices has increased in recent years and there has been a corresponding increase in community placements for student nurses. This chapter introduces the principles of community-based health promotion work including health needs assessment, patient and public involvement and community development. It challenges nursing students to consider whether they can move from a more expert-led, authoritarian role to one that encourages patients and the public to be more involved in the determinants of health – personally and in their community.

Learning outcomes

By the end of this chapter you will be able to:

- define community and why it is an important setting for health workers
- describe the difference between community-based practice and community development
- discuss community involvement and community development and apply it to nursing practice.

Working in communities

Some nurses work *in* communities in primary care. These nursing roles are varied and include posts such as health visitor, community nurse specialist, school nurse and district nurse. The roles vary from providing one-to-one clinical care to teaching sexual health in schools to running breastfeeding drop-in centres. Many of these roles have changed in the past decade and have moved towards a public health role with more of a population focus. One key document that reflected these changes is *Saving Lives: Our Healthier Nation* (DoH 1999a) which identified one group of nurses, health visitors, as public health practitioners with a key role in achieving this strategy by working in collaboration with local agencies, local communities and PCTs. The report suggested that health visitors could conduct more community-based programmes and work with local communities to identify needs. It proposed the following health improvement activities:

* child health programmes
* parenting support and education including support to Sure Start, parenting groups and home visits
* developing networks in communities, e.g. tackling social isolation in older people
* support and advice for breastfeeding mothers and women at risk of postnatal depression
* health promotion programmes to target cancer, coronary heart disease (CHD) and stroke, accidents and mental health
* advice on family relationships and support to vulnerable children and their families.

Activity

Find a copy of your local newspaper. List the kinds of community groups mentioned. Are they run by professionals or by community members?

What do the types of groups listed tell you about the community?

The types of groups listed in the papers will differ from community to community. However, the type of groups included will show what ethnic groups live in the area and give an indication of the age groups that predominate. It might also indicate the types of faith groups that are active in the area and in some cases the health concerns or social issues. In addition to giving some insight into the community, this is also a useful means of identifying the regular groups that meet in order to work with them to deliver services or education sessions instead of trying to set up new ones.

Defining 'community'

Nurses work with communities and patients who are members of many communities and they need to understand communities and how to work with them. They also need to identify how to assess the needs of these communities. In order to gain a full understanding of what this means, it is necessary to define 'community', which is not an easy thing to do.

Activity

Think about the communities that you are part of.
What are they?
What communities do you work with?
Think broadly about this term community to include groups that
    you belong to.

Community has been defined in a variety of ways ranging from very specific definitions to others that are broad and general. Some suggest that the term is used in so many different ways that it is a meaningless term. However, the notion of community has such a crucial role in consideration of community health that it is too important to be rejected (Wass, 2000).

The World Health Organization (WHO) defines community in the following way.

> A specific group of people, often living in a defined geographical area, who share a common culture, values and norms, are arranged in a social structure according to relationships which the community has developed over time. Members of a community gain their personal and social identity by sharing common beliefs, values and norms which have been developed by the community in the past and may be modified in the future. They exhibit some awareness of their identity as a group and share common needs and a commitment to meeting them (WHO, 1998).

As the WHO definition states, communities are often defined as groups of people in a particular geographic location or when the term is used to refer to society, as a group of people or population. However, other definitions are more dynamic, for example, defining community as a 'living' organism with interactive webs of ties among neighbourhoods, organisations, friends and families. These definitions emphasise that they are social systems, bound together by either shared values or shared interests.

Implied in these definitions, is the notion of participation in the life of the community and identification as members of the community. This leads to a sense of belonging which may be described as 'a sense of community' (Wass, 2000). If the definition of community is limited to the idea of a shared geographical location, it may ignore communities of interest.

Activity

Individual patients are part of groups and communities. Think about a patient on a ward that you have seen lately.
What groups or communities did s/he belong to?
What were the beliefs and behaviour of those groups or communities?
Were any of the groups considered to be excluded from society or the health care system?
How were they excluded and why?

These might include groups of single parents, new mothers and people with the same chronic health condition, religious groups or people interested in certain social or environmental movements, to name a few. These communities may share beliefs about their health and ill-health and the ways in which they make health decisions. For example, the Mens Health Forum (www.menshealthforum.org.uk) exists to ensure that health services and policy take account of 'the specific experiences and needs of men and boys'. Yet communities and groups are not necessarily homogenous – although Black and minority ethnic groups have higher than average health and social care needs, there is a substantial variation in the health status of ethnic groups. It is important for the nurse to recognise difference and diversity but at the same time avoid stereotyping especially on the basis of supposed cultural differences. One way to avoid this is to work with groups and communities to identify their needs.

Needs assessment

The term 'needs assessment' is used to describe a process of gathering information that will give a good indication of the priority needs of a community. The process may illustrate the level of poverty or deprivation, access to services, occupation, age, gender and/or social class of the population. It provides a starting point of baseline information from which to measure progress and achievement (Wright, 2001).

According to Stevens and Gillam (1998) there are three approaches to assessing need: epidemiological, corporate or stakeholder and individual. They suggest that doing a three-pronged approach gives a more comprehensive view of a community's needs.

The **epidemiological approach** has been discussed in detail in Chapter 6 and will only be described briefly here. This method of needs assessment provides factual data on the distribution and determinants of health and illness in a population or community. It can help show the type of health issues, the scale of the problem, the natural history of the problem, the distribution of the issue (ages, ethnicity, locality) and predisposing conditions or risk factors. It sets the stage and gives an overview of health and illness in a population.

The second of these is the **corporate or stakeholder approach**. This method involves asking key agencies, service providers and health professionals about the types of health issues and services in the community. Through this approach, needs can be assessed from a professional perspective looking at service provision and gaps. Whilst this is a limited perspective, it is helpful in looking at the health needs of a community.

The **individual approach** is one that has often been neglected in health care provision as the experts have often determined what the needs might be. The method is critical in finding out what the community and people feel are their most pressing needs and how to address them.

When undertaking a needs assessment, it is important to consider that needs will be thought of differently, depending on who is consulted. Needs are sometimes classified as:

- normative needs
- felt needs
- expressed needs
- comparative needs.

Normative needs

These are needs based on the opinion and experience of experts according to current research and findings, e.g. health experts consider that there is no safe level of tobacco smoking. Therefore, a primary health care provider may strongly advise a client who is a smoker to quit smoking. Another example might be a nurse identifying that a patient is obese by calculating a body mass index (BMI), and therefore will advise the patient on the health risks of being obese and on weight loss strategies.

Felt needs

These are things that groups or individuals say they want, or the problems that they think need addressing. For example, the community is demanding more access to fresh fruit and vegetables in their area at a reasonable price.

Expressed needs

These are shown by the number of people using community facilities and services. For example, waiting lists for childcare may express a need for more childcare centres.

Comparative needs

These are shown by comparing what is available to one group of people with what is available to another group. For example, one PCT provides a mobile sexual health service for young people and the neighbouring PCT requires young people to access a genitourinary medicine (GUM) clinic in a hospital.

Needs assessment can provide an opportunity for the community to become involved in the planning of services and programmes from the beginning. It also helps with allocating resources and making decisions about where to start with health promotion work.

There are many ways to find out about a community's needs and assets. One way might be to organise a survey at the school gates to find out what parents want. Another might be to knock on doors to see what people's concerns are about the area they live in. Each of these methods has benefits and limitations. All methods should be planned systematically in order to get a cross section of views from that community and to ensure that not just the loudest or most confident members are heard from.

The main methods of doing a needs assessment are presented below.

Snapshot approach

This gives a quick picture of the needs of the community, in the shortest time period using the least resources. The planners choose practical methods of eliciting people's views, the findings are reported and action on the findings happens quickly.

Questionnaires

Questionnaire design is a highly skilled task. There are advantages of using them as they can reach large numbers of people and are anonymous. The disadvantages are problems with design, asking the right questions, ensuring that the respondents can read them and the inability to explore issues in any depth. The return rate is often very low, which means the results may not be representative of the community.

Focus groups

These are group interviews which focus on particular topics or issues. They are useful in evaluation and can allow the opportunity to explore issues in more depth than questionnaires. However, planning is a key to ensure the groups are representative.

Interviews

This is a verbal one-to-one method. These allow for exploring topics or issues in depth. They can be structured (rigid questions prepared in advance) or semi-structured (allowing for more probing of questions) or unstructured. These are very time consuming and skills are needed to do them well.

Storytelling

This is a qualitative method of gathering information which uses stories as ways of conveying information. It engages others and provides human points of contact that cause people to reflect on their lives.

Participatory appraisal

Participatory appraisal (PA) takes a whole community approach to action research. It uses a variety of tools, techniques and exercises. It consists of three parts: research, education and collection (Henderson *et al*, 2004).

Sharing the results of the needs assessment with the community is a key part of the planning process. This process will:

- raise community awareness about the issues and possible underlying causes
- stimulate discussion about ways to address the issues
- get the community more involved in planning and decision-making about the project

The following scenario provides an example of using an informal needs assessment to find out what the community wants thereby moving to a more participatory means of practice.

Scenario

Helen is a community nurse working in primary care in a large urban area in the UK. Her work involves providing educational opportunities for expectant and new mothers to ensure that they have the knowledge and skills necessary to give their children a healthy start in life. Many of these parents are considered 'at-risk' because they live on a housing estate in a deprived area where they face barriers to good health such as low income, social isolation and limited employment skills.

Participants meet every week. At the end of each class, participants identify the topics they want addressed at the next session. In response to their information needs, Helen covers topics such as the birthing process, breastfeeding, healthy eating during and after pregnancy, smoking, drugs, alcohol, healthy child development, making baby food, and parenting skills. To ensure that participants have adequate resources to meet their nutritional needs, Healthy Start (food and milk) vouchers are provided. The program also provides access to childcare so participants can attend the classes.

While the women were satisfied with the classes, there was a growing concern that other important health issues in the community were not being addressed. Over time, discussions held during the classes focused on other barriers to health faced by participants and their families, such as a lack of recreation facilities for young children and a shortage of affordable day care spaces. While many of the women expressed their need to get a job and support their families once their children were old enough, they were concerned that barriers such as a lack of proficiency in English and a lack of job training programs in the community would limit their ability to do so.

In response to the needs expressed by participants, Helen contacted several community service agencies in the neighbourhood. She collaborated with the other agencies to organise a community-wide forum at one of the community centres. This event resulted in the formation of an inter-sectoral committee made up of agency representatives and community residents.

Over the next two years, the committee pursued activities in response to the needs and priorities identified by community members. These included:

- one of the Sure Start programmes providing parents with access to computers so they could develop resumes and upgrade their computer skills

Continued

- a successful proposal for funding which allowed a local day care centre to offer free half-day 'play-days' twice a week for children aged 2–4 years
- residents successfully lobbying the council to clean and upgrade playground facilities in two housing estates
- the local library expanding its story telling program to include local language stories every week
- the committee organising fun days as a social event for community residents during the summer
- Helen's agency setting up an education and support group for new fathers

What features of health promotion are evident in Helen's practice?

Adapted from: Ontario Health Promotion Resource System (2005)

This scenario incorporates the key features of health promotion practice and community involvement in health issues, including:

- **a holistic view of health** that went beyond the physical health status of new and expectant mothers and children to encompass the social and mental dimensions of health and wellbeing
- **a focus on participatory approaches** that entailed the direct involvement of community members in planning and implementing activities in response to their shared health concerns
- a focus on the **determinants of health** through activities addressing the social, economic and environmental factors contributing to health such as employment, recreation, social support, literacy skills, healthy child development and access to childcare
- **building on existing strengths and assets** by making use of existing community resources and facilities wherever possible and building on the capacity of community residents
- using **multiple, complementary strategies** including health education, self help/mutual aid, organisational change, community mobilisation and advocacy.

Promoting health in communities

Health promotion places an emphasis on empowerment and people taking control over their health. Aspects of this shift are psychological and include improvements in a person's self efficacy or ability to do something and their self-esteem. Other characteristics concern group dynamics and refer to improved abilities to support and network in a community. Strengthening the knowledge and skills of the key actors or stakeholders in a community is sometimes referred to as 'capacity building'. Other aspects of community empowerment describe broader social changes in beliefs, political governance and policies, such that there is more equity in the distribution of status, authority, wealth and influence among individuals or groups (Labonte, 1993). Labonte contends that this empowering process is both health promoting in itself and increases groups' and institutions' abilities to act on specific health problems.

Community involvement and participation

The Alma Alta Declaration stated that community participation in health care is essential and that 'people have the right and duty to participate individually and collectively in the planning and implementing of their health care' (WHO, 1978). The release of the Ottawa Charter in 1986 (WHO, 1986) lent further support for the importance of community development or community action as a health promotion strategy. The Ottawa Charter calls for the active role of the public through tangible and effective community action in setting health priorities, making decisions, planning strategies and implementing them to achieve better health. It strongly rejects the notion of communities as passive recipients of health care professional interventions (Boutilier *et al*, 2000).

Over the past few years there has been an increased interest in the use of participatory approaches and in particular their value in improving the health of communities. Patient and public involvement (PPI) has been advocated as a key strategy in the UK in improving health (DoH 1999b) and is central to National Health Service (NHS) policy. The Health and Social Care Act (DoH 2001) places a legal duty on NHS organisations to ensure patients and the public are consulted at the early planning and organisation of services. Other government documents have also echoed support for the PPI strategy as a way of ensuring that services are shaped around the concern and convenience of patients (DoH 2000). In the government policy and practice guidelines *Strengthening Accountability* (DoH 2003) guidance is given on how to engage with patients and the public on their experiences, ideas, suggestions and plans. Some examples of this are:

- patient-centred services, e.g. integrated care pathways
- patients as partners in their own care, e.g. The Expert Patient Programme (diabetes, arthritis, CHD)
- increased accountability of services:
  — patient forums in every PCT to bring the patient's perspective to decision making

— Patient Advisory and Liaison Services (PALS) providing on-the-spot help and advice
— local authority Overview and Scrutiny Committees (OSC) to scrutinise local health services
- the focus on the neighbourhood as setting for health initiatives, e.g. Local Area Agreements.

Activity

List the reasons why you think involving people in decision-making about their own health and health care and the design and delivery of services and programmes is good practice or a good thing to do.

Some of the reasons for involving people in decision-making about their own health and health care and the design and delivery of services and programmes might be that it:

- identifies unmet needs
- enables organisations and health workers to get a clearer idea of what is important to local communities
- improves quality through measuring satisfaction
- enables resources to be targeted effectively and to prioritise future spending
- ensures that services will be used and are relevant for the local context
- encourages greater ownership and commitment to services and projects that they have been involved in designing and may help to restore confidence in public services
- contributes to greater openness and accountability (Naidoo and Wills, 2005).

People might be involved in different ways and the degree of participation may vary significantly. It might be as limited as taking part in a consultation on clinic opening times to more involvement such as being part of a patient user group or running a local food growing scheme in the neighbourhood. Rifkin *et al* (2000) make a distinction between 'mobilisation (getting people to do what professionals think best) and involvement (according to WHO terminology, having people actively decide what they think is best with the role of professionals to contribute to expertise and resources to enable this)'.

Developing local communities

Developing local communities involves working with the communities to identify their needs and to build on the skills and knowledge of community members to enhance or improve their lives as members of the community. Case study 9.1 describes how this was done in Hull with a project called Developing Our Communities (DOC).

Case study 9.1: Developing our communities project in Hull, UK (Hull DOC, 2001)

Developing Our Communities (DOC) started in January 1996 and was funded from a variety of sources including the New Opportunities Fund, NHS Trusts and the Single Regeneration Budget (government funding for economic and social development).

Hull DOC community workers started by getting to know people and the communities by listening to their hopes, aspirations and needs. Each community had different identities and cultures and many factors had an impact on the quality of life. The initial work built trust, confidence and a sense of value and self-worth within the communities. It included outreach to marginalised people so that confidence and learning increased, community networks were strengthened and people felt more able to have a collective voice in decision-making processes. Examples of DOCs work included:

- carrying out a participatory appraisal involving communities in looking at what was going on in the areas and finding ways collectively to improve community life
- community celebrations – bringing people together to facilitate a community event such as community plays, lunches and parties
- community information – developing an interactive website with communities
- meeting people in their locality – community workers have office space in the community and provide facilities and resources to the community; community workers attend group meetings
- creating an informal local reference group so that residents can network, raise issues and prioritise work for Hull DOC. This included nominating people to sit on the 'Community Chest' panel which awards grants to community groups
- food initiatives, such as food cooperatives, developed by the food community workers to increase access to low cost food.

Community development

Community development (CD) is one approach to developing communities which is based on the idea that people in communities already know what the issues and problems are and how to solve them. The CD approach can assist communities to undertake projects in planned and structured ways, acknowledging the skills and knowledge of local people. Hawe *et al* (1990) define CD as the 'process of facilitating the community's awareness of the factors and forces which empower them with the skills needed for taking control over and improving those conditions in their community which affect their health and way of life. It often involves helping them to identify issues of concern and facilitating their efforts to bring about change in these areas.'

Implied in this definition of community development is the notion that the needs, problems or issues around which a community is organised must be identified by the community members themselves, not by an outside organisation.

The community development process for a health promotion project is likely to have the following stages:

- people identifying the problem or issue
- people deciding what to do about it
- people identifying the resources they need
- people doing the work together
- people learning and developing their skills
- people seeing the benefits of their efforts
- people evaluating the results of their work together.

The cycle then starts again with people identifying the problem or issue of concern (Department of Health and Community Services, 1999).

CD is built on core values and based on certain commitments to working with communities. These are listed in Table 9.1.

Table 9.1 Community development: core values and commitments.

Definition	Core values	Commitments
Community development (CD) is about building active and sustainable communities based on social justice and mutual respect CD is about changing power structures to remove the barriers that prevent people from participating in the issues that affect their lives	• Social justice • Participation • Equality • Learning • Cooperation	• Challenging discrimination and oppression • Encouraging networking • Ensuring access and choice for all groups • Influencing policy from community perspectives • Prioritising concerns of people experiencing poverty and exclusion • Promoting long-term sustainable change • Reversing inequality and power imbalance • Protecting the environment

Source: Standing Committee for Community Development (2001)

Using a CD approach involves working together in partnership with others. Partnership implies equal participation – however this is often not the case. Working in partnership means that people take part in deciding what, when and how work will be done. Instead of just being consulted, or asked, people become joint decision-makers – they share power equally (Wass, 2000).

For the individual nurse, CD is challenging because the approach may not be supported and the nurse is likely to be working alone and have a competing case load. Case study 9.2 is an example of a nurse using CD approaches to improve health.

Case study 9.2: Community development approaches to improve health

In the UK, there is increasing awareness of the capacity of community development approaches to improve health. Jane Naish, policy advisor with the Royal College of Nursing, UK, describes one successful project.

Jenny Gough is an experienced public health nurse and health visitor who has worked in a socially deprived area of the UK's West Midlands for several years. She quickly recognised the multiple health needs and very poor mortality and morbidity record in her community relative to adjacent areas. She was also aware that many health problems were not located at an individual level, that is, they were not simply the result of individual behaviour and 'lifestyles', but the result of poverty and life circumstances.

Because she is a nurse, Jenny is trusted and has access to lives and homes within her community in a way which other statutory agencies, such as social services and the police force, do not. The CD project which she founded began by engaging some of the key stakeholders in the community in looking at the problems as they defined them.

Initially a key issue raised by the community was the lack of community-based facilities, especially for families with young children (the area had a high proportion of single parent families). Jenny carried out some small-scale research with single parents on their needs and through this was able to demonstrate to health managers the need to develop further community-based services for families. From this flowed a commitment from some employers and some limited resources. With these resources, Jenny was able to develop a range of initiatives with the community including:

- shopping trips to local markets with mothers followed by cooking skills sessions at the local community centre (Jenny organised the transport and paid for the shopping)

Continued

- breakfast clubs at the local primary school whereby children could arrive early and have breakfast together at school
- a range of family learning activities whereby parents and children learn together, especially around reading and mathematics
- literacy classes including English as a foreign language for women whose first language was not English
- weight management sessions (which Jenny participated in)
- 'drop-in' health sessions at which any member of the community could access Jenny on any health related issue without an appointment or any bureaucratic process.

Much of the day-to-day running of the above activities was later taken over by the community indicating the sense of community ownership of this project and ensuring sustainability. Other aspects of Jenny's project were also very positive. For example, the breakfast clubs, in addition to improving children's nutritional status, led to increased attendance at school and teachers reporting greater concentration and application to learning by the children. In fact, the project was so successful that she was asked to join the Wolverhampton Health Authority public health management team. She is also involved in the 'New Deal for Communities', a UK policy initiative in England which aims to attract local investment into communities including that from private enterprise.

Adapted from: European Public Health Alliance (2003)

In localities, a more strategic approach has been taken to CD work. Healthy Living Centres are an example of this. One successful example is in Bromley by Bow in East London which is described in case study 9.3.

Case study 9.3: The CAN do culture of Bromley by Bow

Every community contains vast resources of human potential and capability, even those communities which seem to have the most problems such as poverty, crime, drug addiction, environmental degradation, loneliness, ill-health and bad housing. Government regeneration programmes have been designed to tackle those problems which need massive public investment (such as poor housing), but there remain all the less apparent problems which are only fully recognised and understood by local people themselves.

One of the most successful examples of a social enterprise or CD approach to tackle the many problems which so often escape the attention of mainstream public services, but which make all the difference to improving the quality of life for people living in the poorest areas is the work of Andrew Mawson in Bromley by Bow in East London. Mawson arrived in Bromley by Bow in 1984, taking over as Minister of the United Reformed Church. He saw the immense problems faced by the local population and put the church's resources of buildings and land at their service. Initially, he offered rooms to a struggling community nursery run by local parents. Other activities followed, including a community care facility working with disabled people, and a wide range of arts projects run by local artists.

Nearly 20 years on, the Bromley by Bow Centre covers a three-acre site, supporting 150 activities each week, and about 35 enterprises are under development. The arts focus has remained strong and has been the basis for many of the enterprises. For example, local artists were offered free studio space in church buildings if they agreed to teach and involve other local residents. Now, Signs of Life brings together practising artists and local teenagers to do community projects (murals, etc.) as well as public and private commissions across London.

Many of the enterprises are run by and for the different cultural groups in the area – there are 50 languages and dialects spoken within ten minutes' walk of the Centre. To give just one example, Zenith Rahman, a local woman, started to tackle the isolation of other Bangladeshi women by setting up cooking and sewing groups. One of these groups is now running the Bandhobi restaurant which provides high quality Sylheti food for community events as well as catering for high profile corporate functions. The other group has become a sewing and craft enterprise.

Zenith has been working at the Centre for over ten years. She is one of many local people who have grown with the Centre. Some started by taking part in activities provided by the Centre, then worked as volunteers and later, as their skills and confidence grew (often as a result of formal training and qualifications organised by the Centre), they were offered paid jobs. The Centre now employs 105 staff and 2000 people pass through the facilities each week.

One of the biggest projects for the Centre has been the development of the first Healthy Living Centre in Britain. This is owned and managed by the community through their own development trust. The Healthy Living Centre offers traditional general practitioner (GP) services (the GP practices pay their rent to the trust), alongside an enormous range of complementary services from counselling to opportunities to work on allotments – which can be a better treatment for depression than a bottle of pills. Bob's Park, which surrounds the Centre, has been transformed by the trust,

Continued

hugely improving the local environment as well as providing jobs (and a boost for the local economy), alongside lots of opportunities for community participation from tree planting to taking on responsibility for community plots in the park. Even the development of the buildings has been carefully managed to ensure the highest quality design and materials.

The attention to detail in Bromley by Bow is a central aspect of everything they do, alongside the focus on encouraging creative and innovative solutions to what are often seen as intractable social problems. It is an entrepreneurial approach, seeking to enable individuals to develop to their full potential through the setting up of business like initiatives which generate money and enterprise. It brings together many well established community action principles of self determination and community enterprise, together with long traditions of philanthropy which aim to ensure benefit for the most vulnerable sectors of society – with more than a dash of private sector entrepreneurial spirit.

Source: British Broadcasting Service (2002)

Activity

Reflect on the examples given for community development.
Can you identify the barriers that might prevent people from working in this way?
How is this strategy different from community-based strategies?

Some of the barriers you might have considered are language and cultural issues, lack of power, lack of skills and confidence, fear, safety and security. In terms of CD strategies, they differ from community-based strategies in several respects. With CD, the problem or issue is defined by the community themselves rather than the sponsoring organisation. The process of planning and implementing the community development initiative is ongoing, based on continual negotiations between organisations and community groups, with the community worker serving as a liaison. CD emphasises enhanced community capacity (e.g., collective problem solving skills), not measurable changes in health risk factors, as the desired outcome.

The role of the nurse in promoting health for communities

The Department of Health document *Liberating the Talents* (2002) states that primary care nurses have a role to play in this changing focus of primary care:

> *Nurses, midwives and health visitors are the largest group of profession-*
> *als involved [in primary care in communities] and will therefore have a*
> *significant impact on patient led and community centred services. Like*
> *any profession their role cannot be described in isolation, and as the*
> *environment becomes more complex and uncertain, they will rely*
> *increasingly on a combination of developing their core skills (both general*
> *and specialist) and membership in multidisciplinary teams and net-*
> *works. Their key attribute will be their ability to fit their skills with a*
> *wide range of others in a way that best meets the needs of the individual*
> *patient or group. They will play to the strengths of their professional*
> *role in integrating the medical and social aspects of health care, promot-*
> *ing self care and crossing organizational boundaries to maximise conti-*
> *nuity of patient care and health improvement.*

There are a number of things that nurses, community health teams and public health staff can do to support a community and enable community action. These include:

- identification of community priorities by conducting a needs assessment
- support of local initiatives that make community residents more able to control and improve their situation
- find out what people know and what they think is important
- share information
- assist with skills development
- assist with research and collection of information.

Moving into the community will require a shift in attitude and ways of working from a focus of practice on the individual to the wider community. According to Wills (2005), CD requires a change in 'mind set' from a task to a community oriented view recognising the individual as part of a larger group or community with specific needs.

Knowing that there are many barriers to CD work but many advantages, the following list provides some suggestions for the nurse to strengthen involvement in CD initiatives. These include:

(1) finding out if the local authority and local voluntary organisations employ community development workers, and arrange to spend time working with them

(2) finding out about local networks and community initiatives such as Local Exchange Trading Schemes (LETS) and how you might contribute

(3) getting involved in local initiatives, e.g. Sure Start programmes, local health improvement programmes, domestic violence forums, crime and disorder partnerships and regeneration initiatives such as New Deal for Communities

(4) undertaking training and professional development to increase your confidence and skills in CD work

(5) looking at creative ways of responding to an unmet need, e.g. healthy eating projects with community dieticians, food coopera- tives, growing food projects

(6) working with existing groups to identify and meet their expressed needs

(7) developing social support networks between families

(8) trying to secure managerial support for this work

(9) documenting your CD work by having a project plan with clear objectives and recording what you do

(10) discussing with public health specialists on the PCT and seeking their support in developing proposals, securing funding and evaluating initiatives.

Summary

This chapter introduced students to the notion of 'community' health promotion and public health work. It has explored the dif- ferences of working with and in communities and how to identify community needs through needs assessment. By exploring the con- cepts of patient and public involvement in health, CD and empow- erment, it has challenged nursing students to consider whether they can move from a more expert-led, authoritarian role to one that encourages patients and the public to be more involved in the determinants of health – personally and in their community.

Further reading and resources

Active Communities Directorate

This organisation contributes to the delivery of objective five of the Home Office's Strategic Plan 2004–2008: 'Citizens, communities and the voluntary sector are more fully engaged in tackling social problems and there is more equality of opportunity and respect for people of all races and religions.' www.homeoffice.gov.uk/inside/org/dob/direct/accu.html

Community Development Foundation

This organisation helps communities achieve greater control over their lives through advising government, supporting community work and carrying out research, evaluation and policy analysis; non-departmental public body sup- ported by the Active Communities Directorate of the UK Home Office. www. cdf.org.uk

Community Health Action

Journal of Community Health UK. Each issue includes articles and reports on community-based health work. www.chuk.org

Men's Health Forum

This is an independent body that lobbies for the development of health services that meet men's needs and to enable men to change their risk-taking behaviours. www.menshealthforum.org.uk.

Paton A. and Higgins V. (2000) Health Promotion in Ethnic Minority Groups. In Kerr J. (Ed.) *Community Health Promotion: Challenges for Practice*. London, Ballière Tindall.

This chapter explores the social policy background from which various approaches to health promotion with ethnic minority communities have grown. The principles of community development are explored and examples of working with ethnic minority groups are examined.

Standing Conference for Community Development (SCCD)

This organisation provides support to local networks through provision of information and networking events. www.com-dev.co.uk. One of their publications is *A Strategic Framework for Community Development* (May 2001).

References

Boutilier M. Cleverly S. and Labonte R. (2000) Community as a setting for health promotion. In Poland B. Green L. and Rootman I. (Eds.) *Settings for Health Promotion: linking theory with practice*. Thousand Oaks, Sage.

British Broadcasting Service (2002) *The CAN do Culture*. Accessed online http://www.bbc.co.uk/education/beyond/factsheets/changing4_prog7.shtml.

Department of Health (1999a) *Saving Lives: Our Healthier Nation*. DoH, London.

Department of Health (1999b) *Patient and public involvement in the new NHS*. DoH, London.

Department of Health (2000) *The NHS Plan: a plan for investment, plan for reform*. DoH, London.

Department of Health (2001) *The Health and Social Care Act (Section 11 Public involvement and consultation)*. The Stationery Office, London.

Department of Health (2002) *Liberating the Talents – Helping Primary Care Trusts and Nurses to Develop the NHS Plan*. DoH, London.

Department of Health (2003) *Strengthening Accountability: involving patients and the public policy guidance*. DoH, London.

Department of Health and Community Services (1999) *Bush Book*. Territory Health Services, Darwin.

European Public Health Alliance (2003) *Nurses take a community approach* (article by J Naish). Accessed online http://www.epha.org/a/569.

Hawe P. Degeling D. and Hall J. (1990) *Evaluating health promotion* (p203). Sydney, Maclennan and Petty.

Henderson P. Sumner S. and Taj T. (2004) *Developing Healthier Communities*. London, Health Development Agency.

Hull Developing Our Communities (2001) *Annual Report* Hull DOC, Hull.

Labonte R. (1993) *Health promotion and empowerment: Practice frameworks*. Centre for Health Promotion/Participation, Toronto.

Naidoo J. and Wills J. (2005) *Public Health and Health Promotion: developing practice* (p110). London, Ballière Tindall.

Ontario Health Promotion Resource System (2005) *Health Promotion 101 – Health Promotion On-line Course*. Accessed online http://www.ohprs.ca/hp101/main.htm.

Rifkin SB. Lewando-Hundt G. and Draper AK. (2000) *Participatory approaches in health promotion and health planning* (p2) London, Health Development Agency.

Standing Committee for Community Development (2001) *Strategic Framework for Community Development*. SCCD, Sheffield.

Stevens A. and Gillam S. (1998) Needs Assessment: from theory to practice, *British Medical Journal*, **316**, 1448–52.

Wass A. (2000) *Promoting health: the primary care approach*. Marrickville, Harcourt Saunders.

Wills J. (2005) Community development in public health and primary care. In Sines D. Appleby F. and Frost H. (Eds.) *Community Health Nursing*. 3rd ed. Oxford, Blackwell Publishing Ltd. pp57–67.

World Health Organization (1978) *Health for All: Alma Alta Declaration*, (p20). WHO, Geneva.

World Health Organization (1986) *Ottawa Charter for Health Promotion*. WHO, Ottawa.

World Health Organization (1998) *Health Promotion Glossary* (p5). WHO, Geneva.

Wright C. (2001) Community Nursing: crossing boundaries to promote health. In Scriven A. and Orme J. (Eds.) *Health promotion: professional perspectives*. Basingstoke, Palgrave Macmillan.

Creating Supportive Environments for Health

Amanda Hesman

Introduction

Health promotion takes place in 'settings' – environments where people learn, work, play and love. Understanding the nature of these settings helps us to understand how to best reach populations and how the setting itself can influence health messages, health approaches and health philosophy. This chapter will explain the origins of the World Health Organization (WHO) healthy settings approach and illustrate the concept with examples from schools, prisons, the health service and the workplace. Within each chosen 'setting', examples of good public health practice will be identified together with the organisational systems needed to create an environment supportive of health, within and between settings.

> ## Learning outcomes
>
> By the end of this chapter you will be able to:
>
> - describe environments that are conducive to health
> - discuss how the nurse and wider inter professional team can contribute to creating supportive environments for health that make it easier for people to make healthier choices
> - discuss how national policy has a local impact in creating supportive environments for health
> - describe the limitations of the settings concept and barriers to its implementation

Creating supportive environments

The Ottawa Charter (WHO, 1986) describes creating supportive environments as a key action for health promotion recognising that an individualistic philosophy to promoting health and wellbeing focuses on the individual, their lifestyle, their risk behaviour and has the danger of blaming the individual for any ill-health. The environmental, socio-economic and social context in which people live creates and maintains individual health behaviours such as smoking as a response to social expectations or drug use as a response to unemployment. The following statement from the Ottawa Charter recognises this interplay between health, context and setting: 'Health is created and lived by people within the settings of their everyday life: where they learn, work, play and love.'

As we saw in Chapter 2 health is determined by the interplay of environmental, organisational and personal factors. The WHO use the term 'settings' to describe environments that can enable health and wellbeing. We all live in such settings whether it be the place we work, the place we live or the place we play. At a national level the following environments have been identified as appropriate health promoting 'settings':

- schools
- prisons
- universities
- hospitals
- workplaces
- local neighbourhoods.

These settings are not merely opportunities for the delivery of health education. A health promoting setting is one that embraces a 'systems' approach towards health. A 'systems' approach towards health is one that addresses (University of Lancashire, 2005):

(1) the creation of a healthy working and living environment
(2) the integration of health promotion and health development into the daily activities of the setting
(3) the development of links with other settings and with the wider community.

Figure 10.1 is adapted from the National Health Service (NHS) Scotland. It shows how health (the tree) has its roots in biological, social and environmental factors. The trunk of the tree is supported by key health promotion principles – participation, equity, empowerment, partnerships and sustainability. The branches of the tree illustrate some of the key activities necessary to promote health in settings, such as policy development, improving the environment, building relation-

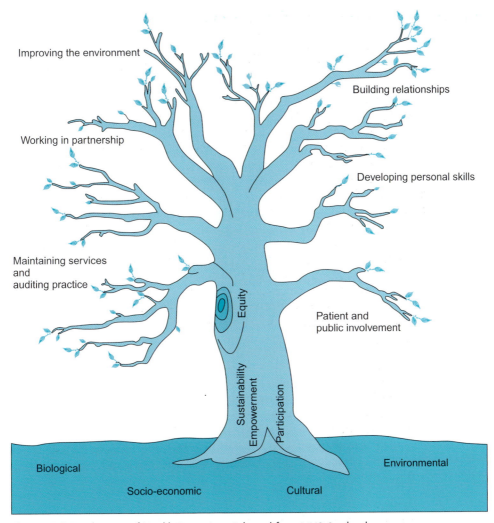

Figure 10.1   The Tree of Health Promotion. Adapted from NHS Scotland.

ships and communication, involving patients and the public, monitoring and auditing services.

Activity

If a central tenet of health promotion is to enable people to take control of their health, to what extent does your work environment enable you to take control of your own health?

To enable a health service setting to be more health promoting requires the practitioner to consider:

- how policies and structures can enable health promoting actions, e.g. a no smoking policy
- how the physical environment impacts on those in the setting, e.g. the ward layout
- how the setting can make partnerships with other agencies and the community to enable it to become more health promoting, e.g. a prison may link with the NHS to promote health
- ways in which individuals can be empowered to take control over their health in the setting, e.g. flexible working arrangements
- ways in which individuals can participate and be involved in determining the shape of the setting, e.g. Patient Advice and Liaison Services (PALS)
- ways in which the setting can contribute to sustainable development and be made more environmentally health promoting, e.g. waste management policies.

Creating supportive environments for health means adopting a wider and more holistic approach that sees health as, 'not merely the absence of disease' (WHO, 1948). An environment can be identified as being supportive to health if it enables healthier choices to be made and therefore sustains healthier living. Case study 10.1 has used the example of cycling as the healthier choice. Cycling has many health benefits not only for the individual but for the environment. Individual health benefits from cycling include increased cardio vascular output, reduced coronary heart disease (CHD) risk factors and maintenance of body weight. At a collective level benefits for the environment include fewer carbon emissions, less traffic pollution, less noise and less congestion (Carnell, 2000).

Case study 10.1: Promoting the health of staff through an integrated transport policy

Policy: cycle helmets are currently VAT exempt. A travel expenses policy may reimburse work related travel by bike such as that adopted by Kings College NHS Trust, London. A health and safety policy will provide additional staff insurance for those cycling to and from work.

Environment: the work environment supports cycling to work with sufficient and secure bike sheds, shower and changing room facilities. The provision of bikes at work that can be used by staff for meetings between sites.

Partnership building: working with local authorities in order to provide training for employees and their families on how to

Continued

cycle safely. Working with local transport planners to ensure that the hospital and surrounding roads facilitate safer cycling.

Empowerment: a consultation exercise that actively seek the views of its employees on barriers to cycling to work and then consults on an action plan to overcome these barriers.

Participation: having a cyclists' user group that informs management of the needs of those cycling to work, for example Newham Trust London has such a group. In conjunction with the Police and transport planners organise a 'critical mass demonstration' for your local area.

Sustainable change: in order to bring about sustainable change cycling to work needs to be the easier choice for the majority of employees, this means prioritising the needs of the cyclist above those of the car driver.

Two useful questions to ask when scrutinising a setting could be:

(1) How *does* this setting currently facilitate health?
(2) How *could* this setting facilitate health?

The answers to the above questions identify where and how health is approached within the setting. This would determine to what extent the ethos of the environment is supportive to health.

Activity

Using these two questions consider the importance that your current work environment puts on healthier eating?
How *does* your work setting currently facilitate healthy eating?
How *could* your work setting facilitate healthy eating?

You may have thought about the type of food provided in the staff canteen and the provision of special diets for patients who are nutritionally deficient, but did you think about your lunch break? Do you get a sufficient lunch break that empowers you to have a nutritious lunch? Are there sufficient staff on duty to assist a patient to be positioned comfortably before meal times, to establish their food preferences and to feed a patient slowly? If you answered 'no' to these last two questions then your work setting does not really sustain healthy eating.

Consider the approaches to health promotion outlined in Chapter 4. The 'settings' approach is one that suggests that action should take place at the socio-environmental level. Table 10.1 compares an 'individual approach' with a 'settings approach' within a given context.

Table 10.1 The settings approach.

Individual approach	Settings approach
• Individual seen as responsible for health	• Setting is seen as responsible for health
• 'Top down' approach	• 'Bottom up' approach
• Agenda set by the organisation or health worker	• Agenda set by individuals through collective action
• Problem lies in individual behaviour	• Problem is within setting
• The setting is passive in the solution	• The setting is active in the solution
• The aim is to control individual behaviour	• The aim is to change the setting and to bring about structural change
• The setting is a vehicle for health education	• The setting becomes health enabling
• Informed by theories such as psychology	• Informed by policies that focus on organisational systems
• Methodology includes mass media, health counselling, behaviour modification programmes, skills development for health	• Methodology includes policies that change organisations, structures and systems
• Topics are health and risk specific	• Focus is on community action and empowerment to enable people to make healthier choices
• Policies focus on topic area	• All policies fundamentally related to health and wellbeing
• No cross cutting policy and limited acknowledgement of systems and processes	• Full acknowledgement of systems and processes

The spectrum of health promotion responsibility can be seen as if on a continuum – at one end the health problem and solution so that the health problem lies with the individual and their behaviour. At the other end of the 'Solution Spectrum' the health problem and solution lie within the setting. Figure 10.2 is a diagrammatic representation showing how public health/health care promotion can be framed.

For example, traditional approaches to tackling workplace stress tend to see the individual as unable to manage the stresses and demands of the job and thus offer counselling and stress management programmes. A 'settings' approach locates the problem clearly in the organisation itself in workplace cultures that inhibit decision-making or control and the solutions might be improving communication strategies or task work groups. The 'health promoting' activity that is utilised will depend on how the problem is framed.

The settings approach

The Ottawa Charter has informed all subsequent recommendations and guidance surrounding the 'settings' approach – its first key action

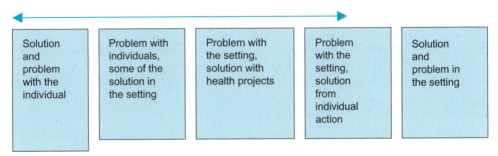

Figure 10.2 The Solution Spectrum. Adapted from Whitelaw *et al* (2001).

area (see Chapter 2) being to enable a supportive environment for health (Poland *et al*, 2000). The European Health for All policy Health 21 (WHO, 1998) also gives direction to the 'settings-based concept'. As a result there have been a number of 'settings' initiatives in the UK and because health is created and maintained outside of the NHS these initiatives encompass a range of environments. Below are some examples of national policy that support the 'settings' agenda and which provide a framework for the implementation of environments supportive to health.

- DoH (2004b) *Choosing Health: Making Healthier Choices Easier*: reinforce schools and the workplace as enablers of health.
- DoH (1998) *Saving Lives: Our Healthier Nation*: refers to healthy homes, schools, workplaces and neighbourhoods.
- DEE (1999) *National Healthy Schools Standard*: actively promotes the settings approach in schools.
- DoH (1999) *The National Service Framework for Mental Health*: standard one promotes mental health in specific settings.
- HSC (2004) *Strategy for Workplace Health and Safety in Great Britain to 2010 and Beyond*: promotes health and safety in the workplace.

A health promoting health service

The Government White Paper *Choosing Health* (DoH, 2004b) has set up a clear role for the NHS in becoming a health improvement service and making the most of the millions of contacts that the service has with people every week to promote health. 890 000 people for example consult a general practitioner (GP) or practice nurse each week; 122 000 people attend as out patients and; 44 000 attend accident and emergency. The social responsibility role of the NHS is also highlighted. It has a huge impact on local economies as an employer and purchaser, with a spend on food and goods and services that represents 10% of regional economies. It also impacts on the environment both as a producer of waste but also in terms of the car miles it demands – NHS staff, patients and visitors in England and Wales travelled an estimated 25 billion passenger kilometres in 2001. Of these, 21 billion (81%) passenger kilometres were travelled by car and van.

The hospital setting

Traditionally hospitals have adopted a 'down stream approach' to health and have only been curative environments for patients. This has meant that hospitals have lacked an emphasis on sustaining and improving health and wellbeing for staff, patients and the wider community. The WHO Health Promoting Hospital (HPH) Network was launched in recognition of the impact that the hospital can have on the health and wellbeing of its staff, patients and the wider population. International policies in support of the HPH include The Budapest Declaration on Health Promoting Hospitals (WHO, 1996) and the Vienna Recommendations on Health Promoting Hospitals (WHO, 1997). In appreciation of the wider public health role that hospitals can have in tackling the broader determinants of health The European Network of Health Promoting Hospitals was launched in 1990 and subsequently the English Network of Health Promoting Hospitals and Trusts was established.

Apart then from improving the quality of care delivered, hospitals can contribute to the health of the population as follows:

- firstly, hospitals exist within a community and an HPH should be establishing alliances and partnerships with their community to promote 'concepts of cure, care and prevention' (Wright *et al*, 2002). For example:
    - promoting and facilitating an osteoporosis prevention programme for the local community targeting women at risk of developing osteoporosis
    - actively seeking user representation from minority and disadvantaged groups such as the intellectually impaired
    - ensuring meaningful involvement from the community when new services are planned
    - provide free first aid training for child minders and parents
    - provide free falls prevention training for elderly groups
    - allow local groups to use hospital premises for meetings
- secondly, as a major source of employment the NHS is ideally placed to improve the health of the local population through health and safety measures at work and via sustainable terms and conditions of employment. For example:
    - implementing healthy working initiatives such as promoting a healthier workplace by providing exercise facilities or offering subsidised membership to local sports facilities

— implementing health and safety policies such as control of substances hazardous to health regulations (COSHH) and no lifting policies
— supporting individuals back to work after periods of sustained illness
— providing a comprehensive occupational health service
— supporting staff in career development
• thirdly, HPH has the potential to work with the local community to lobby and influence local and regional policy on issues such as:
— transport planning
— road traffic accidents
— smoke free environments
— provision of healthy catering in private and public care homes
— 24 hour drinking
— access to affordable, high quality fruit and vegetables.

Case study 10.2: Lancashire teaching hospitals NHS trust

The staff restaurant at Lancashire Teaching Hospitals NHS Trust offers a range of healthy eating choices, with special promotions including free breakfasts to cyclists during Bike to Work Week and, during Bowel Awareness Week, the offer of free fruit to everyone who buys a meal. A fitness and leisure club scheme in Lancashire offers staff discounts at local health clubs – and a hospital-based welfare rights team is being established for patients, visitors and staff, in partnership with Lancashire County Council. The trust's green transport policy includes discounted bus tickets, secure bike stands, another project with the County Council to develop hospital site and local route maps for cyclists, a car sharing scheme and the loan of pedometers to encourage people to walk to work. Other initiatives include a Citizens Advice Bureau telephone advice service – on offer nine hours a week – and a new arts and mental health programme involving patients and visitors in the design of stained glass panels for a central staircase linking ward areas. The idea is to raise awareness of mental health issues and engage individuals and organisations in the use of arts in health care.

Source: Millar (2003)

Activity

Debate the following: 'health services are designed to deal with health' or 'health services are designed to deal with illness' Which statement do you agree with and why?

The reality of the hospital setting is one that has many barriers to improving the health and wellbeing of staff, patients, visitors and the local population. These include financial, physical, organisational and motivational.

- **Staff**: lack of readily available lifting equipment, poor standard of induction programmes for new members of staff, poor communication and consultation procedures, poor supervision of learners.
- **Patients**: high rates of hospital acquired infection that delay recovery, long periods of unnecessary immobility, insufficient information on their condition, prognosis and progress, insufficient hydration, insufficient pain relief.
- **Visitors**: unduly restrictive visiting times, insufficient signposts on hospital grounds, poor access by public transport, expensive or lack of car parking facilities for high priority users.

Case study 10.3 provides an example of how good public health practice can be utilised in the hospital setting to reduce the acquisition of hospital acquired infections (HAIs). A significant amount of HAIs are avoidable and can cause avoidable harm for example methicillin resistant *staphylococcus aureus* (MRSA) has been involved in 0.2% of all deaths in NHS general hospitals (ONS, 2005). The National Audit Office in 2000 published estimates that HAI was a primary factor in 5000 deaths a year and contributed to 15 000 more (NAO, 2000).

Case study 10.3: Promoting the health of patients by reducing the incidence of MRSA

Policy: local implementation of evidence-based and achievable 'protective health policies' such as infection control policies and screening policies for those identified as being at high risk of having MRSA.

Environment: ensure the promotion of health with adequate hand washing facilities and availability of alcohol hand rub for staff, patients and visitors. Ensure staff have sufficient uniforms and adequate changing facilities. Availability of side rooms when indicated by risk assessment.

Partnership building: with the local media to ensure accurate reflection of the situation without 'scare mongering'. Staff should be able to communicate to patients and visitors an accurate account of the risks and how the risk can be managed. Ensure that frontline staff are able to influence ward infection control policy.

Empowerment: empower health care workers by ensuring they have relevant knowledge and skills and health education to

Continued

include transmission, prevention and treatment including their role in preventing antibiotic resistance. Skills include effective hand washing and the ability to communicate the difference between colonisation and infection.

Participation: with the local population and patient groups by involving them and keeping them informed of any action plan and change in incidence rates. Empower patients to challenge poor practice, e.g. when hands have not been washed and aprons not changed between care delivery.

Sustainable change: to bring about sustainable change means for good practice to be maintained.

An HPH as well as involving staff in any change process, be it a change in practice or a change in service, will also involve patients. The NHS Improvement Plan puts the patient at the centre of decision-making about their health. Patients are experts in their health care and have a great deal of experience and knowledge about their needs and local services (DoH, 2004c).

Activity

Think about how service users and relatives can be involved in a collaborative and meaningful fashion to improve care and treatment. Make a list that includes examples obtained from your local NHS hospital, Primary Care Trust (PCT) or prison.

Two examples to get you started are patient panels and carers' groups.

Patient and public involvement should be an everyday occurrence in service delivery in every health setting. However the reality is that patients do not feel listened to and staff can be scared of patients and the wider implication of involvement. Staff involved in service commissioning and service delivery need to be trained on how to engage with expert patients and communities. Health teams can work towards patient friendly accreditation in order to demonstrate commitment to patient involvement (4Ps, 2006).

The pharmacy setting

Community pharmacists are an essential partnership within the health promoting health service and are in an ideal position to promote the health and wellbeing of their local community as they see over 90% of the population per year (Anderson, 2000). Pharmacists see healthy and ill people and may have established relationships and rapport with many of their regular customers. Regular customers will include those people with long-term conditions such as diabetes and CHD and those that have physical and intellectual disabilities that require pharmacological support and advice on health management. Pharmacists are considered experts on medicines by health workers and the public alike, which puts them in an influential position to promote health and prevent ill-health.

Pharmacy services that focus on health prevention include:

- advice on immunisations and vaccinations
- chlamydia screening
- access to emergency contraception
- identification of individuals that would benefit from 'over the counter' statins.

Pharmacy services that focus on health education include:

- medication concordance, adherence and the management of poly pharmacy
- advice on the management of long-term conditions such as asthma
- participation in media campaigns such as Medicines Awareness Week, how to deal with the flu and the taking of folic acid in pregnancy
- skills training, e.g. inhaler technique for people with asthma
- advice on methadone programmes and benzodiazepine reduction
- symptom management
- local knowledge of statutory and non statutory health services.

Pharmacy services that focus on health protection include:

- smoking cessation programmes that use nicotine replacement therapy and behaviour modification intervention
- ensuring antibiotics are prescribed appropriately and by actively participating in the monitoring of antibiotic prescriptions
- ensuring that the pharmacy is accessible in location, has appropriate opening times and has an atmosphere that facilitates open communication
- pregnancy testing.

Activity: How pharmacy services support people with long-term conditions

Investigate your local pharmacy.
   Find out what support and advice they can give to someone with an established long-term condition such as diabetes?

An individual with diabetes may benefit from secondary or tertiary health interventions, discussion of lifestyle changes, management of poly pharmacy and referral to a long-term condition management programme such as the Expert Patient Programme (EPP). Reasons for non concordance with medication are varied and may include lack of understanding, lack of information, fear of side effects, 'feeling better', denial of need and an attempt at regaining some autonomy. Evidence indicates that participation in self-management programmes does increase a sense of empowerment and symptom control. There are two national structured educational programmes for diabetics – Diabetes Education and Self Management for Ongoing and Newly Diagnosed Diabetics (DESMOND) aimed at type 2 diabetics and Dose Adjustment For Normal Eating (DAFNE) aimed at type 1 diabetics (DoH, 2005).

Although a pharmacy has the potential to promote health there are barriers to its development as a health promoting setting: often a pharmacy may lack a confidential area for discussion; pharmacists do not routinely receive training in health promotion specifically on models of behaviour change; and despite new contractual arrangements to broaden the health improvement role of pharmacies they are nevertheless set up as commercial businesses.

The school setting

The school setting has clearly been identified and supported in national policy as an environment that should be supportive to health (DoH, 2004a). Health promoting schools (HPS) aim to link the day-to-day living of the child in the school to the home and to make education a route to healthy values and beliefs becoming established. HPS can support health by:

- incorporating health issues into classroom teaching, e.g. sexual health and smoking
- school health services, e.g. vaccination and screening programmes
- the physical space and building, e.g. sufficient areas for recreation
- identifying vulnerable pupils, e.g. those at risk from malnourishment
- establishing a network of partnerships within the school, e.g. with catering staff and with the local community and with environmental health officers
- ensuring that policies that impact on staff, pupils and parents have a health framework. Involving parents and carers in policy formulation such as the provision of nutritious meals may also impact on their own health promoting behaviour.

Schools fully involved with the National Healthy Schools Standard (NHSS) find that their standards improve faster than the national average with the most demonstrable evidence to be found in schools from areas with the highest levels of deprivation.

HPS that meet the NHSS are expected to demonstrate a whole school approach showing how the school tackles:

- personal, social and health education including sex and relationship education and drug education (including alcohol, tobacco and volatile substance abuse)
- healthy eating
- physical activity
- emotional health and wellbeing (including bullying).

Activity

By using the following three approaches – 'health prevention', 'health education' and 'health protection' (see Chapter 4) consider how the school setting can make healthier choices easier.

Try and give three examples for each heading.

The school setting for health prevention:

(1) implementing a 'walking bus' to reduce the school run by car and increase exercise
(2) —
(3) —
(4) —

The school setting for health education:

(1) teaching assertiveness skills in order for pupils to make healthier decisions
(2) —
(3) —
(4) —

The school setting for health protection:

(1) ensure adequate and freely available drinking water to prevent dehydration and aid concentration
(2) —
(3) —
(4) —

The prison setting

Prisons may not be immediately identified as a setting to promote health but the significant health problems experienced by prisoners demand a health improvement role. One health needs assessment found 'a high incidence of mental illness. In any one week 50% of the prison population suffer neurotic disorders and 1 in 10 suffer psychotic disorders. Suicide is eight times more common among prisoners and 1 in every 60 prisoners self harms. Half of prisoners are heavy alcohol users, 80% are smokers, half are dependent on an illegal substance and at least one quarter have injected drugs' (WHO, 2004). In general there is a poor standard of health care in prisons and staff morale is low as is professional development (Joint Prison Service/NHS Executive Working Group, 1999).

The majority of prisoners have experienced major problems prior to incarceration to a far greater extent than the general population. These include (ONS, 1998):

- debt
- exclusion from school
- dismissal or redundancy
- running away from home
- relationship breakdown
- homelessness
- bullying
- death of a parent or sibling
- violence at home
- serious illness/injury
- sexual abuse.

These problems do not resolve during imprisonment and their psychological effects may become exacerbated during incarceration or upon release. The situation is compounded by being in prison adding to the sense of isolation and hopelessness. Socio-economic deprivation is also over represented in the prison population and dispersal to different prison settings can add to the feeling of loneliness particularly in those people who do not have the right to remain in the UK and do not speak English.

Activity: The prison nurse and the promotion of health

What partnerships and initiatives could the prison nurse be involved in to improve mental health and wellbeing of clients and staff?

The prison has been identified internationally (WHO, 2003; WHO, 2004) and nationally in *Health Promoting Prisons: A shared approach* document (DoH, 2002) as an environment that needs to be supportive for health. The Prison Service Order for Health Promotion (PSO3200) gives advice on how to put into practice this guidance and focuses on the following health issues (DoH, 2003):

- mental health promotion
- healthy eating and nutrition
- healthy lifestyles including sex and relationships and active living
- drug and other substance use.

A health promoting prison (HPP) will need to consider such health problems as part of an integrated rehabilitation programme that addresses communication and life skills and educational and employment development in preparation for release. This integration should encompass interdisciplinary working.

In 2002 the responsibility for health policy moved from the Home Office to the Department of Health. Now PCTs have been made responsible for the commissioning of prison health services within their locality and these should be evident in their Prison Health Delivery Plans that should have been informed by a Health Needs Assessment (HNA).

Two major constraints to promoting health and wellbeing in a prison exist. Firstly, prisoners do not appear to be given the same standard of care and opportunities to access that care compared to those not imprisoned and secondly, a degree of tension exists between a desire for the appropriate level of security and the need for a positive health promoting environment.

The role of the nurse in creating supportive environments for health

The nurse can contribute to the health promoting environment in three ways:

- as a nurse giving direct patient care which includes promoting and sustaining behaviour change
- as a responsible employee
- as an active citizen.

It is necessary for the nurse to recognise their contribution to health and wellbeing as a member of an interdisciplinary team and to be conscious of their role and responsibilities in respect to the setting's core values. A nurse is, of course, responsible to individual patients and clients but needs to remain mindful and be critically aware of the 'bigger picture' and reflect upon how they can contribute to the health setting's philosophy. Aspects of the 'bigger picture' that the nurse needs to actively reflect upon and contribute to include the following:

- **policy**, e.g. implementing health and safety legislation
- **environment**, e.g. identifying physical barriers to care for people with sensory impairment
- **partnership building**, e.g. understanding and respecting the different roles within the interdisciplinary team
- **empowerment**, e.g. ensuring that patients and their relatives know about the PALS
- **participation**, e.g. seeking out service user views
- **sustainable change**, e.g. making sure changes are to systems and thus sustainable.

The nurse is able to contribute towards an environment supportive of health both directly and indirectly. Health and wellbeing can be sustained and improved upon whilst participating in direct individual care and indirectly by contributing to the settings philosophy.

Summary

This chapter has discussed the settings-based approach and its underpinning principles. Settings-based health promotion has a particular philosophy that focuses on 'whole systems' with particular emphasis on participation, partnerships internally and externally, the physical environment and structures. A health promoting setting is also one that becomes 'an advocate for developing healthy public policy at both local and national level' (Dooris and Thompson, 2001). Yet often the root causes of ill-health that arise from the setting are not addressed and the setting is simply a delivery site targeting interventions at the individual rather than the setting itself. The settings approach provides a practical way to think about health promotion within specific settings such as hospitals, prisons, pharmacies, neighbourhoods, workplaces and schools. The intricacies of such large organisations provide challenges that can limit the potential for improving health and wellbeing.

Further reading and resources

4Ps: http://www.4Ps.com. A specialist development agency working to implement the Patient and Public Involvement agenda in health and social care. The 4Ps assessment criteria are designed to help you develop patient friendliness.

www.4Ps.com

DAFNE: http://www.dafne.uk.com

DESMOND: http://www.desmond-project.org.uk/. This is a national education programme for type 2 diabetics.

Health in Prisons Project (HIPP, 2004) *Promoting Health in Prisons – A good practice guide*: http://www.hipp-europ.org.

The Expert Patients Programme: http://www.expertpatients.nhs.uk/. This is a self-management course giving people the confidence, skills and knowledge to manage their condition better and be more in control of their lives.

Ubido J. Winters L. Ashton M. Scott Samuel A. Atherton J. and Johnstone F. (2006) Top Tips for Healthier Hospitals. Liverpool, Liverpool Public Health Observatory/Cheshire and Merseyside Public Health Network. Available online http://www.nwph.net/champs/Publications/Top%20tip2%20for%20h ealthier%20hospitals%20-%20FULL%20report.doc.

University of Lancashire Healthy Setting Development Unit: http://www. uclan.ac.uk/facs/health/hsdu/theory/theoryintro.htm.

WHO Centre for Health Promotion in Hospitals and Health Care: http:// www.hph-hc.cc/mission.php.

References

Anderson C. (2000) Health promotion in community pharmacy: the UK situation, *Patient Education and Counselling*, **39**, 285–91.

Carnell D. (2000) Cycling and health promotion, *British Medical Journal*, **320**, 888.

Joint Prison Service/NHS Executive Working Group (1999) *The Future Organisation of Prison Health Care*. DoH, London.

Department for Education and Science (1999) *National Healthy Schools Standard*. DfES, London.

Department of Health (1998) *Saving Lives: Our Healthier Nation*. The Stationery Office, London.

Department of Health (1999) *The National Service Framework for Mental Health*. DoH, London.

Department of Health (2002) *Health Promoting Prisons: A shared approach*. Crown Copyright, London.

Department of Health (2003) *The Prison Service Order for Health Promotion (PSO3200)*. HMS Prison Service, London.

Department of Health (2004a) *The NHS Knowledge and Skills Framework*. The Stationery Office, London.

Department of Health (2004b) *Choosing Health: Making Healthier Choices Easier*. The Stationery Office, London.

Department of Health (2004c) *NHS Improvement Plan 2004: Putting people at the heart of public services*. The Stationery Office, London.

Department of Health (2005) *Improving Diabetes Services: The NSF Two Years on London*. DoH, London.

Dooris M. and Thompson J. (2001) Health-promoting Universities. An Overview. In Scriven A. and Orme J. (Eds.) *Health Promotion Professional Perspectives* 2nd ed. Basingstoke, Palgrave Macmillan/Open University.

4Ps (2006) *Patient Friendly Accreditation and Assessment.* Accessed online www.patientfriendly.org.uk.

Health and Safety Commission (2004) *Strategy for Work Place Health and Safety in Great Britain to 2010 and Beyond.* Accessed online http://www.hse.gov.uk/aboutus/plans/index.htm.

Millar B. (2003) In Sickness and In Health, *Health Development Today*, **15**, 26–8.

National Audit Office (2000) *The management and control of hospital acquired infections in acute NHS trust in England.* NAO, London.

Office for National Statistics (1998) *Psychiatric morbidity among prisoners: summary report.* DNS, London.

Office for National Statistics (2005) *Deaths involving MRSA: England and Wales, 1993–2003.* ONS, London.

Poland B. Green L. and Rootman I. (2000) Settings for health promotion: linking theory and practice. London, Sage.

University of Central Lancashire Healthy Settings Development Unit (2004) *A new dawn for settings?* Lancashire, University of Central Lancashire.

University of Lancashire (2005) *Health settings theory overview.* Accessed online http://www.uclan.ac.uk/facs/health/hsdu/theory/theoryintro.htm.

Whitelaw S. Baxendale A. Bryce C. Machardy L. Young I. and Witney E. (2001) 'Settings' based health promotion: a review, *Health Promotion International*, **16**, 4, 339–52.

World Health Organization (1948) *Constitution.* WHO, Geneva.

World Health Organization (1986) Ottawa Charter for Health Promotion. *Health Promotion*, **1**, 4, i–v.

World Health Organization (1993) *The European Network for Health Promoting Schools.* WHO, Copenhagen.

World Health Organization (1996; 1997) *WHO Collaborating Centre for Health Promotion in Hospitals and Health Care.* Accessed online http://www.hph_hc.cc/home.php.

World Health Organization (1998) *Health 21 – the WHO European policy for health for all in the 21st century.* WHO, Copenhagen.

World Health Organization (2003) *Prison Health as a part of Public Health.* WHO, Copenhagen.

World Health Organization (2004) *The Health in Prisons Project in Lisbon 1996.* WHO, Copenhagen.

Wright J. Franks A. Ayers P. Jones K. Roberts T. and Whitty P. (2002) Public Health Hospitals. The missing link in health improvement, *Journal of Public Health Medicine*, **24**, 3, 152–5.

Index